Body, Mind & Health

A Biblical Approach to Wholeness

by Monte Kline, Ph.D.

Published by:

Pacific Health Center

PO Box 1066

Sisters, OR 97759

www.pacifichealthcenter.com

ISBN-13:978-1503303935

ISBN-10:1503303934

Copyright 1992 by Monte L. Kline

PUBLISHER'S NOTE: The information contained in this book is not intended for diagnosing illness or prescribing treatment. Rather the material herein is designed to be used in cooperation with your health practitioner to deal with personal health problems. Should you use this information on your own, you are prescribing for yourself, which is your constitutional right, but neither the author nor the publisher assume responsibility.

Table of Contents

Appendix A – Physical Health: A Health Strategy for Anyone . . . Anywhere

Appendix B – Emotional & Spiritual Health: Encounter God through Personal Retreats

Introduction

Your Health Checklist

Examine yourselves . . . (II Corinthians 13:5)

> *"Mr. Kline, you have cancer, and we need to operate immediately."*

So, began my adventure into discovering God's health and wholeness, an adventure that continues over forty years later. I had thought I was whole – I was a Christian, in vocational Christian ministry, 24 years young, married with a new baby. Everything *should* have been okay, but that simple statement from a doctor revealed how "unwhole" I really was.

Maybe that's your story as well. You have health problems or may even be in a health crisis right now. Even worse, you just don't know why. You think you're doing the right things for your health, but something must be missing. Is there some magic drug or vitamin that would solve all your problems? Probably not. But there is another way of approaching health – a way to discover what's missing in your health "recipe." That's what this book is about.

What is health anyway? Is it just "the absence of disease" as I was taught in junior high school or something much more? The answer to that question is found in the word itself: Health comes from the old English word *hale*. Guess what other word also comes from "hale?" It's the word **whole.** Therefore, to be healthy is to be whole. So what then does it mean to be "whole?" Most people think of wholeness and health only in terms of the physical body. But that's only one-third of who we really are. The Bible reveals that God made us three-dimensional people – body, mind and spirit. To possess wholeness in all three dimensions is the real definition of health. Unless you are experiencing God's design for body, mind and spirit, you lack wholeness and health will elude you.

Have you ever walked into a shopping mall looking for a particular store (or maybe the restroom)? If you're like me, you probably look for that big mall map near the entrance showing where everything is and containing three very special words:

YOU ARE HERE

To go anywhere you must first know where you are – what is the starting point? Self-examination tells you where you are, and in so doing, is fundamental to all areas of life. When it comes to health, not everyone has the same needs. Some people have a lot of "missing ingredients" in the physical dimension but may have things together pretty well emotionally and spiritually. Others are very physically healthy, but void of any spiritual life. Still others may be emotional and psychologically healthy, yet "out to lunch" in the other two dimensions.

Recognizing this problem, I developed a "Checklist for Health" – a self-evaluation tool for measuring your physical, emotional and spiritual health. It simply lists some of the major ingredients for health for body, mind and spirit. Though the rest of this book will give a more detailed examination of these aspects of health, for the moment we only want them as a checklist. If you are mostly practicing that item, check it off – it's not likely to be a cause of health problems for you. However, if you are mostly *not* practicing it, leave it blank. The blanks that you cannot honestly check off reveal what's missing in your "health recipe."

CHECKLIST FOR HEALTH

Body

_____ I primarily eat a diet of whole, natural foods.

_____ I regularly go through a cleansing/detoxifying program.

_____ I do aerobic exercise three or more days per week.

_____ I drink purified water rather than tap water.

_____ I spend some time outside daily getting fresh, pure air and sunlight.

_____ I take high quality nutritional supplements according to my nutrient deficiencies.

Mind

_____ I generally love myself – I have a positive self-image.

_____ I usually look at the positive side of my circumstances.

_____ I am free from guilt over past or present failures.

_____ I generally feel love for other people.

_____ I accept people who have different views from mine.

_____ In relating to another person I am more interested in experiencing a positive, loving relationship than in just being "right."

_____ I forgive others who wrong me rather than holding resentments or anger.

Spirit

_____ I have a relationship with God through faith in Jesus Christ as my Savior from sin.

_____ I have surrendered the control of my life to the lordship of Christ.

_____ I have discovered and resolved spiritual strongholds affecting my life.

_____ I see God's grace expressed on the cross completing all my deficiencies

_____ I am trusting God to sovereignly work through my

circumstances to fulfill his purposes for my life.

THE "HOLES" IN YOUR WHOLENESS

What could you check off? More importantly, what couldn't you
check off? The later represent the *holes in your wholeness*!
Conversely, the areas you easily checked off represent your areas of
greater strength and maturity. Don't be fooled by the simplicity of
the checklist. The ingredients of health really are pretty simple for
the most part. The problem is that we like to make health more
complicated than it really is. Plus, we just plain avoid self-
examination, preferring to just keep too busy to reflect on where we
really are. We'll do just about anything to keep from truly examining
ourselves as the Bible commands.

Few people lack all the ingredients of body, mind and spirit health.
Usually we tend to "camp" in a given dimension while minimizing
the others. I don't know how many people I've met over the years
that were "into health," as far as diet and taking vitamins, but really
weren't very healthy at all in the overall "body, mind and spirit"
sense. They had holes in their wholeness. Sometimes they were
ignoring physical ingredients like detoxification. They were trying to
solve every health problem with another vitamin pill when their
body *first* needed cleansing. More typically, though, they lacked in
the emotional or spiritual areas – areas for which no vitamin pill will
suffice. But that doesn't stop many people from trying.

I could tell a lot of stories at this point. Many years ago I met a well-
known health food "guru" whose focus was on raw food. Eating
everything raw was the answer to all your health problems. I will
never forget how offended she was when I expressed the opinion
that her health problems primarily resulted from emotional stress
rather than nutritional deficiencies. She thought I was a heretic for
suggesting such a concept! And, by the way, this person was a
Christian and *should* have known health was about a lot more than
just the physical.

Let me share another story that typifies this problem: When I was first in clinical practice, a semi-retired couple traveling in a motor home came into our clinic for testing. Since our testing instrumentation could electronically evaluate the compatibility of nutritional supplements, the lady wanted me to test the products she had, as is pretty routine in my practice. What isn't routine is the two large boxes of vitamins she then brought in with perhaps 50 bottles of vitamins! Naturally I queried her about why she was carrying so many vitamins (most of them unopened, by the way) around the country with her in their motor home. Her reply was typical:

> *I read a lot of articles and hear a lot of programs about different vitamins. Every time I learn about something that is supposed to help a problem I have, I go out and buy it.*

What was she doing? By trying to solve all her health problems with just limited physical remedies, she was ignoring a lot of other health ingredients. I must admit, I spent much of my life doing the same thing, trying vitamin and vitamin to solve my health problems, often going from one "fad nutrient" to another, always hoping the next vitamin pill I would try would be the answer:

> *Well, zinc is supposed to be good for that – I'll try it*

> *Funny, that didn't work; maybe I need selenium. No, that didn't help either*

> *Oh, it must be aloe vera that I need." "Gosh that didn't work.*

> *Maybe a raw food diet will straighten me out.*

And on and on it goes – a futile attempt to achieve total health using only physical ingredients of health. If you've ever wondered why you see so many sickly people at health conventions (and I mean the ones that have been involved in doing all the "right" nutritional things for years), I submit that this is the reason. The song talks about "looking for love in all the wrong places," but a lot of people are looking for health in all the wrong places too.

Don't misunderstand me. I'm not criticizing taking nutritional supplements. I take a lot of nutritional supplements and suggest supplements for my clients. Any particular supplement or diet may help certain people for whom it is appropriate. But if you have that area covered already, if you've already devoted a lot of attention to properly nourishing your body, you'll usually find the answers to your remaining health problems somewhere other than in a vitamin bottle. The point is to **evaluate** which dimensions of your health are lacking and then supply those deficiencies, whether they are physical, mental or spiritual.

But now let's get into the specifics of health in body, mind and spirit. What are the physical, emotional and spiritual ingredients that will make us healthy, that will make us whole? And more importantly, how do we supply those missing ingredients?

Chapter 1

God-Made Food

Listen diligently to me, and eat what is good. (Isaiah 55:2b)

A dentist friend of mine shared a story of the mother of one of his patients whom he found particularly frustrating. The child suffered from numerous dental and other health problems, and Mom couldn't figure out why. In a moment of wisdom he gave some simple advice to her saying:

> *If you want to fix his health problems, stop feeding him man-made food and start feeding him God-made food.*

Could it really be that simple? Absolutely. I must ask you the same question: Are you eating man-made food or God-made food?

It's not news to say that food is essential to life. But which food is that "God-made food" that will produce optimum health in your body? It seems everyone has a different idea about what's good to eat and what isn't. "Scientific" studies and professional opinions muddy the water even more: One study says coffee's bad; another says it's good. One authority is for meat; others push vegetarianism. One opinion tells you to eat unsaturated fats; another says they give you, rather than prevent heart disease. And on it goes. How do you navigate this turbulent sea of opposing ideas about food and health?

Have you ever pondered the significance of God giving man instructions on eating immediately after the creation? We read in Genesis:

> *And God said, "Behold, I have given you every plant yielding seed that is on the face of all the earth, and every tree with seed in its fruit. You shall have them for food."* (Genesis 1:29)

But, before you renounce meat and go vegetarian based on this verse, don't stop reading at the first chapter of the Book. God had more to say about food *after* the flood:

> *Every moving thing that lives shall be food for you. And as I gave you the green plants, I give you everything. But you shall not eat flesh with its life, that is, its blood.* (Genesis 9:3-4)

The fallen, post-flood world was no longer vegetarian, whether out of necessity, physical changes in the earth or unknown reasons. But the story further unfolds in the food restrictions in the Dietary Law given by Moses:

> *This is the law about beast and bird and every living creature that moves through the waters and every creature that swarms on the ground, to make a distinction between the unclean and the clean and between the living creature that may be eaten and the living creature that may not be eaten.* (Leviticus 11:46-47)

But was this "word" on food again changed in the New Testament? I'll come back to that question a little later. My point for right now is simply that God, in his goodness, has repeatedly spoken about his provision of food for life and health. The question is whether or not we are listening.

"MAGIC" EATING

Surely most people believe there is something "magic" about eating. How else can we explain people filling their bodies with "foodless food" and expecting no health consequences? Deep down, most people think that whatever they eat (as long as it tastes good and is filling) will be magically transformed into a healthy body. Even the alchemists of old, trying to turn lead into gold, weren't that crazy! Is it really logical that you can eat a sugar-covered, deep fat fried donut with no consequences? Where exactly in the gastrointestinal tract does the "magic" happen that transforms the donut into nutrients that feed and build and repair your body?

To think about it another way, would you pour water in your gas tank and expect your car's engine to magically transform that water into the proper fuel? I mean, after all, isn't one liquid as good as another? Get ready for engine failure and a lot of repair expenses! Or would you "water" your garden with your gasoline can expecting the dirt to change the gas into water? That would be absurd. Or how about using aluminum rods instead of plutonium in a nuclear reactor? What's the difference? Aren't they're both metals? But isn't that what most of us really believe about food? We seldom have any fear or hesitation of the consequences of using the wrong fuel for our bodies.

The famous GIGO (garbage in – garbage out) expression originated with computer programmers, but it captures the issue of food and health as well. What you put into your body is what you get by way of result. Do you really want a healthy body? Then put good stuff into your body? There's no "magic" – just simple cause and effect that follows from the choices you make.

FOOD VS. "FOOD PRODUCTS"

If I opened your refrigerator and kitchen cupboards, would I find food or just "food products?" Just because something is marketed as "food," that doesn't make it so. Food is simply the God-made items provided to nourish our bodies, while "food products," though they often start from food, are man-made through refining and adulteration with additives. To put it another way, food that didn't exist 100 years ago is not food – it's just a food product that was never designed by God to go into your body. Beware of the marketplace which constantly pitches new "food products." Real food hasn't changed.

PROVISION VS. PERVERSION

I have a principle that explains food, and a lot of other things in this world:

God Provides – Man Perverts

God Creates – Satan Counterfeits

God is a perfect provider for all our needs – physical, emotional and spiritual. Read what the Psalmist says about God's perfect provision of food:

> *You cause the grass to grow for the livestock and plants for man to cultivate, that he may bring forth food from the earth and wine to gladden the heart of man, oil to make his face shine and bread to strengthen man's heart. (Psalm 104:14-15)*

But what do we do with his perfect provisions? We often pervert them into something harmful. To put it another way, God is a perfect Creator, but our adversary, the devil, counterfeits good creation with death-producing imitations. James wrote:

> *Every good thing bestowed, and every perfect gift is from above, coming down from the Father of Lights, with whom there is no variation or shifting shadow.(James 1:17)*

Whatever "good and perfect thing" God has created and provided, fallen man manages to utterly ruin:

Wealth to Greed

Love to Lust

Sex to Illegitimacy and Disease

The Environment to Pollution

Fire to Destruction

Healthful Food to Junk Food

DEAD FOOD

So let's talk about what man has done to food. God-made food is:

Living, whole and pure

while man-made food is:

Dead, refined and adulterated

So, what is "living" food vs. "dead" food? You probably *hope* your food is dead before you eat it, so what are we talking about? Think about the history of a tomato I go to the store and buy. After being grown with chemical fertilizers, it was picked green many days before to allow for transport and storage. That results in a lower nutrient value than that fruit *would* have had through natural ripening. Storage time is always the enemy of nutrition. The longer that tomato sits in a rail car, warehouse, delivery truck or supermarket bin, the more nutrition is lost. To add further insult to injury, we then cook the poor thing to death bringing further loss of its food value.

Contrast that with the fully ripe tomato I just picked from my garden and plopped into my mouth. The taste alone tells the whole story. That ripe tomato is delicious, while the supermarket tomato tastes like wet cardboard. That ripe tomato from my garden is a *living* food, while supermarket tomato is a *dead* food. I define a *living* food as one that is eaten as close in time as possible to its life source. Pick it ripe and eat it – it's still living. Pick it green and transport it and store it for days (or weeks), and it's dead.

REFINED FOOD

 Man-made food is also "refined" as opposed to being "whole." Refining refers to removing certain parts of a whole food, usually to make a more palatable or less perishable food product. Sugar cane is a great example. Whole sugar cane is rich in a number of vitamins and minerals, but when it is refined into white sugar, no vitamins or minerals remain. God created foods must be eaten whole, rather than fractionated by refining, since his design has purpose for *every part* of a given food. The sugar refining process removes the B vitamins naturally found in sugar cane, preventing the proper metabolism of sugar. In fact, research done by John Yudkin, MD in England, shows that refined sugar actually leaches nutrients from the body stores. It's what nutritionists call an **anti-nutrient** – the more sugar you eat, the more deficient in nutrients your body becomes. Provision or perversion? Creation or counterfeit?

Whole grains, such as whole wheat, provide yet another example. Again, I would emphasize that *all* the parts of the grain are there for the Creator's purposes. When we have all three parts – the bran, the germ, and the endosperm – we have a wonderful God-made food. However, refining into white flour removes the bran (the fiber) and the germ – the very parts containing the most nutrition. That leaves only the endosperm, which is the starchy part of the whole grain. Low fiber, white sugar and white flour diets are now implicated in many, if not most, of the degenerative diseases of so-called "civilized" countries. Provision or perversion? Creation or counterfeit?

3 "WHITES" -- SUGAR, FLOUR & SALT

We might round out our "three whites" of man-made food with white salt. Sea water contains 84 minerals in about the same concentration as in our blood serum or amniotic fluid. For millennia living sea water was air and sun dried into unrefined sea salt for the preserving and flavoring of food, not to mention its value as a perfect trace mineral supplement. This is the salt you read of in the Bible.

But then along comes salt refining. It begins with rarely using sea water for salt, but rather using mined salt from inland areas. What's the difference? The sea water is a living system, while salt from a mine or ancient lake bed is dead. Refining then reduces salt down to just two minerals – sodium and chloride – creating a totally unnatural, dead and refined food product that may taste about the same even though it is a perversion and counterfeit of the original.

High heat processing *kills* the salt, removing 82 of the 84 minerals found in sea water *refines* the salt, and the addition of harmful additives to prevent moisture absorption and caking *adulterates* the salt. Regarding this last step in the making of this man-made food, the most commonly used additives are aluminum compounds, which have been associated with Alzheimer's disease and other conditions. Corn sugar (dextrose) is likewise a common salt additive to keep the salt free-flowing. This is just what you need – **sugar added to your salt!**

Does it seem strange that so much effort is expended to refine the goodness out of salt? Why go to all that effort and cost to produce an essentially unhealthy product? Here's the dirty little secret: Only 7% of the sodium chloride salt that is refined goes for food uses, while the other 93% goes to industrial uses. Pure sodium chloride is a common chemical reagent used in the manufacture of explosives, chlorine gas, soda, fertilizers, and plastics. Since the manufacturer's objective is primarily to produce sodium chloride for industry, scant concern is given to its toxic effect on human biology.

But there's more: What do think happens to those other 82 minerals refined out to make plain sodium chloride? Because those trace minerals are quite valuable, they are sold to generate significant income for the manufacturer. Real salt is perverted and counterfeited into a man-made food simply because most people won't notice the difference. Refined sugar still tastes sweet, refined flour still is filling, and refined salt still tastes salty with only two of the original 84 minerals remaining.

SO-CALLED "SEA SALT"

Many people think they've solved the salt problem by buying "sea salt" at their health food store. For all practical purposes most of what is labeled "sea salt" is essentially the same as regular white table salt. It is refined and bleached salt that is 98%+ sodium chloride. All that the name "sea salt" means is that it came from sea water. Whether you refine sea water or mined salt down to just sodium chloride, you still have a dead and refined food product. However, there are a few unrefined, air and sun dried sea salts containing all 84 minerals found in sea water. A special preserve off the Brittany Coast of France features this historic salt farming, which produces products such as Celtic Sea Salt (pronounced **kel**-tic with a hard "c"), a product used in my practice for many years.

ADULTERATED FOOD

Thirdly, man-made food is "adulterated" instead of "pure." While refining refers to taking the good stuff out of natural foods, adulteration refers to putting bad things into the food. This is the realm of food additives – over 10,000 chemicals added to our foods to:

Extend shelf life

Enhance appearance

Enhance taste

In other words, food additives (as well as food refining) mainly serve an economic benefit to the food product manufacturer.

The entire philosophy behind food additives reeks of arrogance against the Creator. It is based on an assumption that there's something wrong or inadequate about the food that God provided that needs a chemical fix by man to kind of straighten it out. However, the problem with these chemical additives is simply that they are not food! Because they weren't created for human consumption, your body treats them as foreign invaders. Is it any wonder that food additive after food additive over the years has been found to cause cancer? Just as you wouldn't dream of contaminating your car's gasoline with sugar, salt, BHA, BHT, MSG, sodium benzoate, dyes emulsifiers, artificial flavors, and the like, why do it to your body? Want a simple rule for good health? Try this:

Add nothing to the food God provided and take nothing away.

HEALTHY FOODS

With all the explanation of dead, refined and adulterated food, some people get the mistaken idea that there's nothing out there fit to eat. Fortunately, that isn't true. Understand that in a fallen world there is no perfect food nor any perfect anything for that matter. We have the opportunity and ability to make better choices, to choose wisely. Many times in my 30 year career as a Clinical Nutritionist, I've had people say things like:

I can't avoid sugar; it's in everything!

Well, excuse me, but it's *not* in <u>everything</u>. Likewise, food additives are not in *everything*. Defeatism is the last refuge of the lazy. If you want to be healthy, it's going to take some effort. You have to educate yourself about food, you have to actually read labels, and you have to think about your food choices instead of just responding in zombie fashion to TV commercials. You can *eat* healthier and *be* healthier.

By way of disclaimer, let me say that the ten good foods I'm highlighting here are *generally* good for *most* people. There are exceptions. You may be sensitive to a particular food, such as wheat, for example. Even though whole wheat is a nutritious food, your allergic sensitivity could produce fatigue, digestive, emotional or other negative symptoms. In such a case your body requires desensitization before you can handle that particular food.

Similarly, particular foods may be contraindicated during particular health problems at a particular time. For example, if your body is particularly toxic and in need of cleansing, concentrated foods like meats and eggs would at least *temporarily* need to be avoided. Or, if you're diabetic, raw honey is probably going to provoke undesirable blood sugar spikes just as refined sugar would. So again, these are *general* guidelines. Consultation with your nutritionally-oriented health professional will address the specifics for your condition.

The ten foods listed below are not the *only* healthy foods. However, they are foundational and historic foods, all of which are spoken of favorably in the Bible. These are the basics that definitely were considered foods not only 100 years ago, but also thousands of years ago. Compare this list with what you eat, and you'll known whether you're really eating **food** or just **food products**, whether you're eating **God-made food** or **man-made food.**

#1 WHOLE GRAINS

Give us this day our daily bread . . . (Matthew 6:11)

Whole grains are perhaps the most foundational food mentioned in the Bible. Jesus described himself as "the bread of life" (John 6:35) in reference to his provision of salvation. Bread represents his body in the Lord's Supper. Old Testament sacrifices used grains (Exodus 29:2; Leviticus 2). It's safe to say that from a biblical point-of-view, grains hold the central position for human nutrition.

Few foods are more nutritious than whole grains – they literally are the "staff of life." By whole grains I am referring to such foods as whole wheat, whole rye, triticale (a wheat-rye cross), buckwheat, brown rice, oats, millet, barley, and spelt. So what makes these basic whole grains so good for us, anyway? Let's take whole wheat as an example. Of the 40-plus essential nutrients recognized, all but six are found in whole wheat. Wheat has a high protein content for all but one essential amino acid – lysine.

Because grains are seeds, they are a concentrated nutritional storehouse capable of producing a new plant – that is, they are a "living" food. Whole grains are very versatile as well – grind them into flour for baking, cook them for cereal, or sprout them for salads. However you happen to use them, once you switch to whole grains, you won't again settle for their refined counterparts.

Now for my caution: Food sensitivities to wheat (or gluten in grains) and to baker's yeast (used in making bread), are extremely common. Although whole wheat is great from strictly a *nutritional* point-of-view, it will be bad for individuals that are sensitive to it. If you are sensitive to wheat, yeast, or any other food for that matter, you may experience fatigue, indigestion, or various other reactions to eating it. Thus, in my practice, we always test people for food sensitivities to prevent such reactions.

Let me also clarify some terminology that is often confusing. I'm talking here about "whole wheat," which refers to the complete grain – bran, germ and endosperm – as compared with white flour, which is only the endosperm (starch) part of the grain. Know that governmental labeling rules define "wheat bread" as bread made with *white* flour. Such bread is sometimes only darker in appearance because of the addition of food colorings. The labeling you're looking for is "whole wheat" or "100% whole wheat."

#2 RAW FRUITS & VEGETABLES

> *. . . I have given you every plant yielding seed that is on the face of all the earth, and every tree with seed in its fruit. You shall have them for food.* (Genesis 1:29)

Raw fruits and vegetables are about as close as you can get to eating food in the form God provided it. In their raw state, close to harvest time, they are "living" foods. While whole grains provide more of the basic fuel to run the body, fruits and vegetables function more to *cleanse* and *repair* the body. Though they are nutritionally "good" even when properly cooked, the ultimate nutritional value of a fruit or vegetable is in its raw state before cooking heat destroys enzymes. Cooking also destroys significant amounts of vitamins, minerals and other nutrients. This creates a problem for canned and frozen fruits and vegetables.

When it comes to fruits, we usually eat them raw, but maybe you haven't discovered raw vegetables. Raw carrots or raw celery are pretty familiar, either eaten alone or sliced or diced into salads. The advent of "salad bars" introduced usage of many other raw vegetables – cauliflower, broccoli, green pepper, sprouts, and others. Perhaps the ultimate of eating raw vegetables would be through raw vegetable juices, with carrot juice or carrot-celery juice being the most popular. Juices are basically a way of getting more concentrated fruits and vegetables. Though these juices can be purchased at health food stores, having your own vegetable juicer is the only way of getting really fresh juices, as well as saving money in the long run.

3 CULTURED DAIRY PRODUCTS

> *For pressing milk produces curds . . . (Proverbs 30:33)*

Contrary to advertising propaganda, milk is not the perfect food for every "body." As a practicing nutritionist I've dealt with thousands who were sensitive to cow's milk, resulting in sinus problems, colds, asthma and other problems. But what does God's creation and God's word tell us about milk, since we're trying to look at foods from that perspective?

First, we would observe that milk is an infant food, not a life-long food:

> *You need milk, not solid food, for everyone who lives on milk is unskilled in the word of righteousness, since he is a child. But solid food is for the mature . . .*(Hebrews 5:12b-14a)

In the creation animals instinctively drink milk only during infancy. Man alone persists in drinking milk into adulthood. The creation would also teach us that the milk of the mother is the only "perfect" food for the baby. Thus, the only baby that cow's milk is a "perfect" food for is a baby calf! Breast milk is therefore the perfect food God designed for human babies.

I would also note that the milk drunk in the Bible is probably not cow's milk, but goat or sheep milk, as is still true in much of the Middle East today. The only uncultured milk I could recommend at all would be goat's milk, in that sheep milk is not generally commercially available. Goat's milk is much more compatible with the human body than cow's milk, but I still wouldn't suggest heavy consumption by adults.

Cultured milk, however, is a whole other story. When we add beneficial bacteria to culture plain milk into cheese, cottage cheese, buttermilk, yogurt or kefir, **we create a different food** that is much more digestible and nutritionally beneficial. Since the enzymes necessary to digest plain milk are not present after infancy, the predigesting effect of culturing the milk largely eliminates that problem. Cultured milks such as yogurt and kefir will actually produce B vitamins by the ongoing action of the bacteria implanted into the intestines. Scientists have found a natural antibiotic value in cultured milks, eight ounces of yogurt reportedly being equivalent to 14 units of penicillin. This in part may explain why most of the very long-lived peoples of the world have some kind of cultured milk in their staple diet.

As in the case of wheat I must make a caution relative to allergic sensitivities. If a cow's milk sensitivity is indicated, even cultured cow's milk products may need to be avoided until the reaction is desensitized. Likewise, cultured milk products may aggravate cold, sinus or asthma problems. Goat's milk products will usually be preferable in such instances, though their usage still requires some caution.

#4 RAW NUTS

> *. . . take some of the choice fruits of the land . . . pistachio nuts and almonds . . .* (Genesis 43:11)

Like whole grains, raw nuts are also seeds containing the necessary life of the plant for its reproduction. Thus, in nuts we have a lot of nutritional benefit in a small package. Nuts are particularly rich in protein, essential fatty acids, B-complex vitamins and other nutrients. I would emphasize that nuts are a concentrated food source, so some people may have difficulty digesting them. Chew them thoroughly and don't overindulge.

Like every other food nuts are subject to the "God Provides – Man Perverts" principle. Few people eat raw nuts as I'm recommending. More commonly nuts are either roasted in oil or dry roasted. Though much nutritional value remains, heating turns raw nuts from a living to a dead food. Oil roasted nuts should particularly be avoided due to trans fats and free radicals associated with heating vegetable oils.

#5 RAW HONEY

> *My son, eat honey for it is good . . .* (Proverbs 24:13a)

With over 60 mentions, it's safe to say that no food is spoken of more highly in the Bible than honey, where it is used as a symbol of wisdom. Raw honey is probably your best bet for a truly natural sweetener, though even the most natural sweeteners should be used sparingly, as also noted in the Bible:

> *If you have found honey, eat only enough for you, lest you have your fill of it and vomit it.* (Proverbs 25:16)

There's more to honey than just being a sweetener. Hippocrates, the father of medicine, prescribed honey to those who wished to live long. He did – he died at 109![1]

Dr. W. G. Sackett, bacteriologist at Colorado State University, found in experiments that every harmful microorganism he introduced into honey died within a few hours.[2] Dr. A Rollender experimented with the blood-building effect of honey at an Austrian orphanage by giving the children two tablespoons of honey per day. Blood hemoglobin levels increased 8 ½ % over the control group.[3] What about fatigue? Going back to ancient Greece, athletes used honey to overcome fatigue. Since muscular fatigue is caused by the build-up of lactic and carbonic acids in the tissues, the alkaline nature of honey, as well as most fruits and vegetables, helps neutralize this.

The health benefits of honey cannot be explained by its rather meager vitamin and mineral content, though. It appears there's something unknown in honey that promotes health. Bodog Beck, M.D. comments:

> *There is no question but what the benefits derived from the daily use of honey cannot be entirely explained by the known elements in honey . . . It is clear that either honey contains vital elements required by the body for health that have not yet been discovered, or else known ingredients are combined in such proportions as to make them more valuable in nutrition than has been realized to date.[4]*

Beware of heat processed honey. The terminology "raw" refers to a lack of high heat extraction of the honey from the comb and fine filtering. Heat extraction would, of course, destroy nutrients, and filtering removes the nutritional value of the pollens that are naturally mixed in with the honey.

#6 UNREFINED FATS & OILS

> *. . . you shall eat the fat of the land.* (Genesis 45:18c)

There's probably more misleading information on the subject of fats and oils in the diet than about any other topic. As a result of decades of "fat bashing" advertisements and promotion of low fat foods, Americans are now experiencing record rates of obesity and other health problems – the very health problems the low fat diets were supposed to cure. I call it "The Big Fat Lie."

When it comes to obesity, the shocking fact is that dietary fat promotes weight loss, but it has to be the right kind of fat. The livestock industry understands this. Feeding pigs polyunsaturated fats like corn or soy oils (the kind we've been told to eat for decades) puts more fat on the animals. To make pigs leaner as slaughter is approaching, the Department of Animal Science at North Carolina State University found it necessary to *stop* feeding polyunsaturated fats and *start* feeding saturated fats like coconut oil. After 30 years of avoiding saturated fats, just like the pigs, Americans have gotten fat.

The Big Fat Lie also extends to cholesterol. Since the late 1950's the "Lipid Hypothesis" was preached to Americans, claiming saturated fat caused high cholesterol which in turn caused heart disease. Yet this was totally refuted by the famous Framingham, Massachusetts study on cholesterol. Contrary to the propaganda we've all been fed, the study found that the more saturated fat people ate, the *lower* their cholesterol!

So what are the good fats? The three I most recommend are these:

1. Virgin Coconut Oil – This is an unrefined, non-heat processed coconut oil, generally imported from the Philippines. As a saturated fat, it is the most chemically stable, not breaking down with heat into harmful substances. This healthy fat's benefits include weight loss, reduction of heart disease risk, cholesterol lowering, energy improvements, skin improvements, metabolism stimulation and help with diseases including diabetes, irritable bowel syndrome (IBS), and Crohn's disease. It is excellent for cooking, baking or even just eating directly in the mouth.

2. Olive Oil – Olive oil is the predominant oil used in the Bible, due to the abundance of olive trees in the Middle East. Olive oil is a monounsaturated oil, which means it is pretty stable and doesn't easily break down into rancidity. Thus, it is also an acceptable cooking oil.

3. Butter – Since publishing my first book in the mid-1970's at the height of the presumed superiority of margarine, I have recommended butter. This was long before the dangers of trans fat in margarine became known. Margarine is artificially saturated fat, while butter is a naturally saturated fat. Margarine is a man-made food; butter is a God-made food. The butyric acid in butter is a short-chain saturated fatty acid possessing anti-bacterial, anti-fungal and anti-viral benefits. It also tastes great!

The conclusion is that we need fats and oils for good health, but they must be the unrefined fats and oils, primarily in the saturated or mono-unsaturated categories.

#7 UNREFINED SALT

> *You shall season all your grain offerings with salt. You shall not let the salt of the covenant with your God be missing from your grain offering; with all your offerings you shall offer salt.* (Leviticus 2:13)

As referred to earlier in the chapter, table salt is a refined, adulterated product with only two elements remaining – sodium and chloride. Unrefined sea salt, such as the Celtic Sea Salt from France, is naturally air and sun dried, just as salt was produced back in biblical times, to contain all 84 elements found in sea water. It produces vast health benefits.

#8 HERBS

> *. . . and the herbs of the mountains are gathered in . . .*
> (Proverbs 27:25b NASB)

Herbs are plants valued for their medicinal, savory, or aromatic qualities. The study and usage of herbs for medicine goes back to the earliest physicians, Hippocrates and Galen. The Bible also makes numerous references to the use of herbs, though the word often translated "herbs" in the King James Version refers to what we would call garden vegetables.

In addition to the medicinal usages of herbs, I see two basic dietary uses for herbs. First is for seasoning food, as we commonly do in our culture with thyme, savory, cayenne, marjoram, basil and other herbs. The second usage would be in the beverage category with herbal teas. Hot herbal teas are a great alternative to caffeine beverages like coffee. Iced herbal teas make an excellent warm weather alternative to carbonated beverages.

#9 FREE RANGE EGGS

> . . . if he asks for an egg, will you give him a scorpion? (Luke 11:12)

Few foods possess the balance and concentration of nutrition found in eggs. While eggs can be an excellent natural food, commercial production methods have greatly compromised their goodness. In a "free range" environment of natural sunlight, eating some grasses, eating insects and "scratching for food" in the dirt, chickens and their eggs are great. Commercially raised eggs are quite different, though. Several birds are crowded into small cages under artificial light and fed hormones to make them pump out as many eggs as possible. Disease is often a significant factor. It doesn't take a college degree to figure out that eggs so *unnaturally* produced won't fulfill God's intended design for food very well.

#10 ORGANIC MEATS

> When the Lord gives you in the evening meat to eat . . . (Exodus 16:8a)

Like eggs, commercially raised meats may pose health threats due to cancer-causing growth stimulant hormones and other drugs. Meats also possess the disadvantage of being near the top of the food chain, resulting in greater levels of environmental toxicity. "Organic meats" refers to animals raised without hormones and other unnecessary drugs. Such a natural environment source for beef, lamb, turkey, and chicken is superior.

Though fresh fish, biblically and historically, is an excellent food, it is becoming increasingly difficult to obtain fish from uncontaminated waters. Most "farmed" fish may present an even greater problem due to feeding practices and increased potential for disease in a crowded environment. My recommendation is to use the best "wild" fish you can, but not too often.

I also strongly urge my clients to abstain from eating the "unclean" animals of the Old Testament Dietary Law, shown by modern scientific research to be toxic and therefore harmful to health.[6] For us it mostly means avoiding pigs, shellfish and other scavenger animals. Understand that there are two aspects to the Dietary Law – a ceremonial aspect and a health aspect as noted in Leviticus:

> . . . *to make a distinction between unclean and the clean, and between the edible creature and the creature which is not to be eaten.* (Leviticus 11:47, NASB)

"Clean" and "unclean" refers to the old covenant ceremonial law which is fulfilled (and therefore abolished) in Christ. But "edible" and "inedible" is talking about something else – health. God did not select the "unclean" animals in some arbitrary fashion. Rather, he essentially said, "I've created some animals for your food and some as garbage collectors, and I want you to know the difference." Just as we are what we eat, so are the scavenger and predatory animals forbidden in the Dietary Law. It only makes sense that their flesh would be unhealthy.

Critics opposing any adherence to the Dietary Law fail to separate its scientifically proven health benefits from its spiritual significance to the nation of Israel. Let me be perfectly clear: There is no spiritual anything associated with following the Dietary Law (or any other part of the Law) today, but there are practical health benefits. Legalism is not about *obeying* the Law, but rather the spiritual significance one attaches to obeying the Law. The same could be said of the Law's prohibition against murder or stealing. The fact that I am not "under the Law," spiritually speaking, doesn't give me license to go out and murder or steal.

The critics often cite various New Testament passages to supposedly prove that Christians shouldn't avoid pig, shellfish, etc. The most common one is Peter's vision in Acts 10 in which the sheet from heaven full of unclean animals is lowered with God saying, "Rise, Peter, kill and eat" (Acts 10:13). Surely this sounds like God wants us to eat every animal, including snakes and eagles and spiders and the like. But this was not Peter's own interpretation of the vision. Rather he said:

> . . . *God has shown me that I should not call any person common or unclean.* Acts 10:28b)

Peter saw the unclean animals of the vision as symbolic of the Gentile nations. As a result, the Jewish believers began preaching the gospel to the Gentiles, beginning with Cornelius. He didn't interpret the vision as permission to serve ham for Sunday dinner! The passage speaks only to the ceremonial significance of the Dietary Law being finished. It does not address the underlying health issues.

When it comes to meat, keep in mind that any form of meat is harder to digest than vegetable sources of protein. Fish is the easiest, and beef is the hardest when it comes to digestion. Therefore, it's wise to restrict meat intake to no more than once per day or even three times per week for optimum health. The biblical usage of meat follows more of this type of pattern. Meat was a special occasion food rather than the three meals per day food it is for most people today. Although meat is a God-made food (given proper raising and absence of contamination), it does require moderation to produce optimum health benefits.

CONCLUSION

Discovering food for life is a matter of looking at God's design as revealed in his word as well as his creation. Instead of eating according to family patterns, culture, or advertising manipulation, we can look for this higher source of wisdom. You might say it's a matter of "following the Manufacturer's instructions." He made an abundance of healthful food for our consumption. Man has unfortunately altered natural food so that it doesn't fulfill its God-intended role. The living, whole, pure food God provided will produce life, health and energy. The dead, refined, adulterated food that man often chooses leads only to fatigue, disease and premature death. The choice is yours.

Chapter 2

Water That Refreshes

For I will pour water on the thirsty land . . . (Isaiah 44:3a)

On November 28, 2009 people in Portland, Oregon woke to the following breaking news:

> *The City of Portland issued a* **boil water notice today** *for the city west of the Willamette River . . . Last week, routine water sampling results from Reservoir 3 in Washington Park indicated the presence of Escherichia coli, commonly known as E. coli. Today, results from a resample of Reservoir 3 water indicate the presence of E. coli in the reservoir . . .*[1]

We take a lot for granted when it comes to water. We turn on the tap and out it comes, just like always. But losing your water supply for a while will change your perspective, like it did for me during a recent sub-zero cold snap at our home when our pump gave out. Replacement took a week – a week of hauling water to horses, hauling water to flush toilets, and showering at our local church. It was an eye opener!

The availability of water, however, is so much more than a mere convenience. Water and life are synonymous, but we prefer to focus more on food as our most important health ingredient. It isn't, and let me prove that. You can go thirty to forty days without food but only a couple of days without water. So which is more fundamental to health?

TWO MAIN ISSUES

Water is about two main issues – quality and quantity. Few people get a sufficient *quantity* of water, but even fewer get a proper *quality* of water. Guess what? Quality doesn't matter if you don't get enough quantity, while quantity doesn't matter if your water is full of poisons. Thus, our goal is simple: resolve both the quantity *and* quality issues concerning water.

WATER QUALITY PROBLEMS

A church I once attended funded several water projects in a remote area of Uganda where people previously relied on disease infested rivers for their supply. That may be the kind of image that comes to your mind when you think of "water quality problems" – third world countries drinking from dirty rivers. Let's face it: In western countries we *assume* water purity. We assume the government is protecting us – an assumption that is an illusion.

Since 2004 testing by water utilities around the United States discovered 315 pollutants in tap water.[2] The majority of these chemicals are not regulated and can legally be in the water in any amount. Recent studies on over 8000 people show higher consumption of tap water increases the risk of bladder cancer in men, but that's only the tip of the iceberg.[3] Few understand the limitations and risk of typical "purification" – limitations that result in numerous kinds of toxic contamination.

SOURCES OF WATER CONTAMINATION

Let's look at the six most common categories of water toxicity:

1. Air Pollution – Wait a minute – weren't we talking about *water* pollution? Air pollution causes water pollution, since the rain and snow fall through the atmosphere. Though I grew up with running water, it was common in our little village in Northern Illinois for people to collect rain water for drinking as an alternative to the hydrogen sulfide "rotten egg" well water from that coal mining area. Once upon a time the water falling as rain and snow was fairly pure, but not anymore.

2. Agricultural Chemicals – Where do all those pesticides, herbicides and nitrates from synthetic fertilizers end up? In the underground water supply of course! For example, the San Joaquin Valley in California has experienced decades of well water contamination from millions of pounds of nitrate fertilizers poured on the ground. But lest we only point our finger at chemical agriculture, I would hasten to add that manure also contaminates the water supply, particularly with the large concentrations of it around feedlots – not to mention your State Legislature or the Congress! Seriously though, chemical *and* organic agriculture both have issues affecting water quality.

3. Industrial Chemical Wastes – There are literally thousands of chemicals in use that may ultimately end up in the water supply. Benzene, trichloroethylene, and thihalomethanes are among the most common.

4. Pathogenic Organisms – In this category we're talking about bacteria, viruses, protozoa, amoebae, and the like. The *Cryptosporidium* protozoan parasite provides a great example with its 1994 outbreak in a major city resulting in 400,000 ill, 41,000 treated, 4000 hospitalized, and 104 dead. This didn't happen in some third world country of Africa, Asia or Latin America, though. The city was Milwaukie, Wisconsin.

5. Chlorination – Wait a minute! Isn't chlorination supposed to be a "good" thing for water purity? Of course chlorination does kill harmful bacteria in water, but, what most people do not know is that it also creates new toxins by combining with organic contaminants. The result is called DHP – disinfection byproducts. Some of the DHP's include chloroform, trihalomethanes (THM's), and haloacetic acid. Research has linked DHP exposure to increased heart, lung, kidney, and central nervous system diseases, not to mention cancer.[4] W. F. Von Deltinger, MD stated that injury to the mitral valve of the heart and cardiac insufficiency may result from severe exposure to chlorine. To add insult to injury chlorine destroys vitamin E, the "heart vitamin."

6. Fluoridation – To say the question of water fluoridation is controversial is to put it mildly. I know of no more incendiary health issue than water fluoridation – even after over 60 years of debate. Pro-fluoridationists have succeeded in portraying anti-fluoridationists as little old ladies that see Communists behind every bush. Actually I know some of those little old ladies fighting fluoridation, and they shouldn't be caricatured. They're smart, well informed, and vigilant against this health scam. As always, personal attacks signal an opponent lacking any good factual argument. Fluoride proponents are masters of propaganda, knowing that if you repeat a lie often enough people will eventually accept it as true. But let's get to the facts.

Fluoridation was originally done with pharmaceutical grade sodium fluoride, an industrial waste that is a byproduct of aluminum manufacture. It should be pointed out that, *prior to water fluoridation,* the primary use of sodium fluoride was for rat poison. The historic scientific studies done on water fluoridation in the late 1940's – the ones proponents always cite as evidence of fluoridation's benefits – were all done with sodium fluoride, a substance seldom used today.

Fluoridation is primarily done now with fluorosilicates and fluorosilicic acid. So what's that? For one thing it's *not* pharmaceutical grade, but comes from the wet scrubbing systems in the stacks at phosphate fertilizer plants. Classified as hazardous waste, it is typically contaminated with arsenic and other heavy metal toxins.[5, 6]

Though many books would be required to discuss the huge amount of scientific research documenting the dangers of water fluoridation, let me mention just a few of those findings:

1. Fluoride is a cumulative poison, that is, it builds up over time in the body. Only half of the fluoride you ingest is excreted through the kidneys.

2. Fluoride readily combines with many metal ions – "good" ions like calcium and magnesium, as well as toxic ions like lead and aluminum. It can interfere with enzymes involving the key nutrient mineral, magnesium, while also facilitating uptake of toxic lead and aluminum.[7]

3. Fluoride may affect brain function. Chinese studies show a lowering of IQ in children exposed to fluoride.[8]

4. Fluoride may create hypothyroidism. Prior to water fluoridation it was common for doctors to use fluoride medications to suppress thyroid function in hyperthyroid patients. Thus, indiscriminant water fluoridation of *everyone's* water has the potential for making normal thyroid individuals low thyroid, potentially resulting in depression, fatigue, weight problems, muscle or joint pains, as well as increased cholesterol and heart disease.[9, 10]

5. Other studies point to increased bone fractures, due to fluoride's effect of making the bones more brittle, not to mention cancer, infertility, and many other problems.

None of these toxic side-effects is really the greatest problem, though. The biggest issue with water fluoridation is the dirty little secret that it does **not** reduce tooth decay, the supposed reason for its existence. Pro-fluoridationists are quick to claim credit for the decline in tooth decay in recent decades but can't explain similar declines in tooth decay where there is no water fluoridation. A survey by the National Institute for Dental Research of 39,000 children from 84 communities show little difference in dental decay rates between those with fluoridated or non-fluoridated water supplies.[11]

We observe the same phenomenon in comparing nations that do and do not fluoridate their water. Though no longer fluoridating water, Canada, Cuba, the former East Germany, and Finland all report similar reductions in tooth decay.[12] Some authorities suggest that the lack of dental decay correlates more with higher income levels than with higher fluoride levels in drinking water.

Again, let me emphasize there is an enormous amount of information on this topic that is beyond the scope of this book. For more information I suggest checking out the Fluoride Action Network at **www.fluoridealert.com**.

WATER PURIFICATION METHODS

Given all the possible pollutants to public water supplies, it's not hard to realize that water is indeed a problem. The question then becomes, "How do I purify my water?" Let's look at several options:

1. Boiling – If you boil water long enough (like for 20 minutes), you will kill bacteria, viruses, and parasites . . . and you'll also make your water a "graveyard" for dead germs. The idea is to **purify** the water, not just kill the bad things in the water and leave them there. Also keep in mind that boiling **concentrates** the solid contaminants, like heavy metals, because they're still there but in less water due to the boiling. Boiling is strictly an emergency method for destroying organism toxins in water when you don't have a better alternative.

2. Rain or Snow Water – As discussed earlier, once upon a time before the industrial revolution and atomic bombs, this was a decent option for water purification, but not today.

3. Well Water – Many people, especially in more rural areas, get their water from a well. Often this will be very pure water, but it depends on many variables – depth, geology, exposure of the surrounding land to agricultural chemicals and manures, and the like. Bottom-line with wells is that you just don't know without extensive testing of the water. Don't presume water quality just because it comes from a well.

4. Filtered Water – Water filters range from inexpensive ones that attach to your kitchen faucet or that you pour water through to expensive solid carbon block filters. Almost any filter will reduce at least some of the chlorine content and eliminate the chlorine odor. For the cheap filters that's about all they do. But even the expensive filters are not effective at removing arsenic, lead, nitrates, parasites, sodium sulfates, bacteria, and viruses. In addition to those limitations the filtering media itself can easily become a breeding ground for bacteria. Any filter is less effective over time – the more water you run through it, the less you are filtering out. Filters are not constant in their degree of toxin removal. Better filters, such as solid carbon block units, have the added disadvantage of high replacement costs.

5. Reverse Osmosis – Reverse osmosis or RO is really just a different type of filtration. An RO unit typically fits under the kitchen sink where it forces water under pressure through a semi-permeable membrane that removes certain toxins. Performance depends upon constant water pressure, so I wouldn't recommend it if you're on a rural well where your pressure varies a lot. I also wouldn't recommend RO if you live someplace where water is expensive, since for every one gallon of purified water you waste six gallons that didn't get through the membrane. Like solid carbon block filters, RO effectiveness decreases over time and the membranes are expensive to replace.

6. De-ionization – This method removes certain organics and dissolved solids well, but doesn't remove pesticides, herbicides, and industrial solvents. As with filters, the resin beds used in the process can become germ breeding grounds.

THE BEST PURIFICATION – DISTILLATION

I have found distillation to be the ultimate purification method, having started using it over 30 years ago after enduring the awful tap water of our Southern California community. Since beginning my clinical practice in 1983, I have exclusively recommended distilled water to my clients. Distillation has a long history of usage by many health conscious people, not to mention the U. S. Navy and cruise ships, both of which derive their fresh water onboard from distillation.

Distillation is not "filtration" of water. In case you forgot your eighth grade science class, distillation refers to boiling a liquid into a vapor and then condensing it back into a liquid form. Combined with post-carbon filtration, where the distilled water is run through a charcoal filter as a final step, this method significantly or completely removes algae, arsenic, bacteria, benzene, chloride, chlorine, fluoride, Cryptosporidium, lead, mercury, nitrates, odors, pesticides, rust, salt, sulfates, and viruses.

Much of my confidence in distillation as a water purification method comes from observing the creation: God has been purifying water by distillation since the beginning. There is no "new" water on earth – we're using the same water that was used by Abraham, Moses, and Jesus. Through a continual process of evaporation and condensation into rain or snow the water on earth is purified.

Another advantage of distillation is its constancy. A water distiller will produce the same purity today as it will six months from now, since turning the liquid into vapor leaves everything behind except the water. Distillers need to be cleaned, but for efficiency rather than for purity.

Dr. Charles McFerrin described the benefits of distilled water this way:

> *Distilled water is "empty" water – a hungry water, a water capable of absorbing body poisons. You have had the experience of trying to use an old post office blotter on the desk. Everybody had used it, and it is so full of ink that it will not suck up any more. So it is with a "full" water, a water full of chlorine, aluminum, etc. Such water does not have the capacity of absorbing body impurities.*

C. W. DeLacy Evans, M.D. in his book, *How to Prolong Life*, claims that distilled water, used regularly in place of spring water or other inorganic mineral water prevents aging by preventing mineral deposits associated with hardening of the arteries:

> *Used as a drink, distilled water is absorbed directly into the blood, the solvent properties of which it increases to such an extent that it will keep in solution salts already existing in the blood, prevent their undue deposit in various organs and*

structures, favor their elimination by the various excreta, and tend to remove these earthly compounds which have already accumulated in the body . . .There is no doubt as to the high value of distilled water used freely as a retarder of the ossifying conditions which appear to constitute the condition of old age.

Dr. Alexander Graham Bell, inventor of the telephone, was a great proponent of drinking distilled water, claiming its daily use had prolonged his life. Afflicted and bed-ridden with sciatica, Dr. Bell could find no relief for the pain. He had read a well-known scientist of the time who stated that old age came from mineral deposits in the system that went uneliminated. Such deposits were said to produce rheumatism, kidney stones, or hardening of the arteries, depending upon where they happened to lodge. When such deposits coated the nerves, sciatica resulted. Bell wrote:

I knew that distilled water was pure. I thought that if I drank plenty of it, I could get rid of some of the salts that were covering my sciatic nerves. I tried drinking it, and it worked like a charm. I have kept up my drinking of distilled water, and I attribute my almost perfect health largely to it.

OBJECTIONS TO DISTILLED WATER

Like most health questions, there is considerable debate on the subject of distilled water. Practitioners I deeply respect hold an opposite view to my own. Nevertheless, most of the objections to distilled water are based on misinformation – myths, if you will:

<u>**Myth #1**</u> – **Distillation removes essential minerals**. The truth is there are no "essential" minerals in water as far as human nutrition is concerned. For example it would take 676 glasses of Boston, Massachusetts tap water to get the Recommended Daily Allowance of calcium, 1848 glasses to get the RDA of magnesium.

Myth #2 – Distillation leaches essential minerals. Critics of distilled water state that it will remove nutrient minerals from your body. This is not only untrue, but it is physiologically impossible for distilled (or any other kind of water for that matter) to extract nutrients from *inside* your cells. What distilled water will do is flush out discarded, unusable minerals that are outside the cells. Improvement in joint symptoms after drinking distilled water is an example of this beneficial effect.

Myth #3 – Distilled water doesn't remove organic chemicals. This statement is both technically correct and wholly inaccurate. Volatile organic chemicals (VOC's) boil at a temperature lower than water. Thus, it is possible for these contaminants to escape the distillation process and end up in the finished distilled water. However, the home water distillers I am familiar with eliminate this problem by (1) having a volatile gas vent (a small hole) at the top of the condensation coil to allow the VOC's to escape and (2) a post-carbon filter the distilled water runs through which likewise eliminates this contaminant.

Myth #4 – Distilled water is acidic. This is basically a false statement, though I'll admit it could be true under certain non-existent circumstances. Distilled water has a neutral pH of 7.0 – it is neither acid nor alkaline. Critics maintain that with exposure to carbon dioxide in the air it becomes acidic. Distilled water is stored in capped jugs without air, so I would question exactly where all this CO2 exposure is supposed to come from. Furthermore, why would distilled water be acidified by the air more than any other purified water (or any water period)? Like most other distilled water myths, this objection is usually perpetrated by those selling competing water purification equipment and has no real basis in fact.

Myth #5 – Distilled water tastes flat. Actually, distilled water has no taste – what tastes is every other kind of water. The universal experience of people who drink distilled water for a while is that they can't stand the taste of any other water. After over 30 years of drinking distilled water, my taste buds are immediately offended by tap water and other so-called "purified" waters. I promise that if you drink distilled water for a few weeks, you'll almost crave it, being unable to stand any other water.

Taste issues with distilled water are normally solved with the post-carbon filtration used on most home water distillers. It definitely will not taste flat. I would add that store-bought distilled water will often have some plastic taste from the container it's sold in, as would any other bottled water. This is another great argument for having your own distiller so you can eliminate possible storage issues.

Myth #6 – Distilled water is expensive. Most store-bought distilled water sells for under a dollar per gallon, though in some places it can cost $1.50 or more. Other bottled waters, of course, have pretty much the same price. However, the cost issue is eliminated by having your own home distiller which will produce a gallon of water for about twenty cents in electricity costs. Thus, a home distiller usually pays for itself in a year or so over the cost of buying distilled water. I have to say, though, that even if my distilled water cost a dollar or two a gallon, it would be worth it in terms of its health benefits, in that nothing is more vital to your health than consuming pure water.

Let me emphasize that if you choose a different purification method from distillation, I won't argue with you. My main exhortation is simple: Don't drink tap water! Any kind of purified water is miles ahead of any tap water. It's just a question of good, better, or best. Whatever water purification method you use, know its limitations. Don't assume it's "taking everything out," because, unless it's distilled with post carbon filtration, it doesn't take everything out.

"STRUCTURING" WATER

In spite of my preceding hearty endorsement of distilled water, I am not without some concerns. Distilled water clearly provides the greatest purity, but there's more to the water question than just purity. Though distillation is God's method of purifying water through the natural evaporation and condensation processes, there is an important distinction – that "naturally" distilled water changes as it falls on the earth, picking up minerals. Well, so what? We've already established that the mineral content of water is *nutritionally* insignificant, but what if minerals in water have another health purpose?

We obviously need distillation to thoroughly remove the junk from water, but shouldn't the water be restored somehow? It's like formatting the hard disk on your computer to get rid of all the corrupted files. You can wipe the disk clean, but you don't have a functioning computer until you restore the good content that should be there. Then, and only then, can you actually *use* your computer. Just as both steps are needed on your computer – erasing and restoring – so, I believe, you need to "erase" and "restore" your water by taking your distilled water to the next step – structuring.

NATURAL WATER STRUCTURING

Let's take an example of naturally "distilled" water falling as rain or snow on the Cascade Mountains that I'm looking out at from my home right now. After falling, that water flows downhill over stones and other objects, forming vortices that oxygenate the water and electromagnetically program it. It bonds with certain minerals that, though nutritionally insignificant, help structure the water molecules resulting in **hexagonal water**.

As we all know water is H_2O – two atoms of hydrogen bonded with one atom of oxygen. But those molecules don't stand alone but rather form structured groups. The healthiest structure involves six water molecules bound together hexagonally. The unhealthiest form features five water molecules bound pentagonally. Certain minerals with stronger chemical bonds decrease the free movement of water and thus encourage the hexagonal structure – calcium, lithium, sodium zinc, silver, nickel, iron, and copper. But other minerals with weaker chemical bonds increase the free movement of water promoting the pentagonal structure – magnesium, potassium, rubidium, aluminum, chlorine, fluorine, bromine, and iodine.

So what will hexagonally structured water do for you? Reported effects include improvement in energy, bone density, obesity, constipation, immunity, and ability to handle stress, among other observations. Water around normal proteins in the body is hexagonal in structure, while water around cancer-causing proteins is pentagonal. Thus, if we want to encourage the healthiest state inside our body, it makes sense to drink hexagonally structured water.

MAKING STRUCTURED WATER

Water may be hexagonally structured by four different methods:

1. Lowering water temperature – Hexagonal structures increase with lowering of the water temperature – thus glaciers are full of structured water. Super cooled water (liquid water below the freezing temperature) is 100% hexagonal in structure. Such a process is not practical unless you happen to live underneath a glacier.

2. Adding structure-making minerals – As previously discussed, certain minerals tend to program the water into a hexagonal structure.

3. Electrical field – An ionization or electrolyzation process is used by placing the water in an electrical field. Positive ions are pulled to one side of a permeable membrane, while negative ions move to the other side. Unfortunately, the resulting hexagonal structure of the water doesn't last long, making this a less than desirable method.

4. **Magnetic field** – A better method uses a magnetic field where the water is spun in a vortex between two opposing pole magnets. With this method the water maintains its hexagonal structure for 20 days. There is also an increased oxygenation effect, but this only lasts about 20 minutes. The most common water structuring appliance uses this method combined with the addition of the hexagonal structure-making minerals.

Structured water can have a powerful detoxifying effect, so some caution is advised when you first begin to use it. It's best to introduce it gradually for the first week or so, before switching to 100% structured water drinking. Beware of detoxification symptoms such as fatigue, achiness or emotional mood changes.

WATER QUANTITY

We've spent a lot of time talking about water *quality*, but we do need to say a word about water *quantity* as well. How much water should you drink? I have to tell you from my experience as a health practitioner that hardly anyone drinks enough water, pure or not, to properly cleanse and detoxify their body. Drinking even the purest water will be of limited help if you don't drink enough of it.

I generally recommend the following rule of thumb: Divide your body weight in pounds in half and drink that number of ounces of pure water per day. For example, if you weigh 128 pounds, you would drink 64 ounces (2 quarts) of water per day. If you weigh 192 pounds, you would drink 96 ounces (3 quarts) per day, etc. Most people are shocked upon hearing this rule of thumb, since hardly anyone drinks that amount of water. But keep in mind that, just through the normal respiration processes, you will lose as much as one to two quarts of water daily, depending upon how warm the weather is. So what happens if you're losing more water than you're replacing through drinking? Ever see a raisin or a dried apricot? That's you!

CONCLUSION

Though often ignored, water is your most important health ingredient. The key is simply getting sufficient quality and quantity of water to cleanse and detoxify your body. Unfortunately we live in a world that doesn't automatically give us pure water. Though you will have to exert some effort and make some investment to get healthy water, the benefits you will experience will make it well worth it.

Chapter 3

Cleansing That Purifies

. . . let us cleanse ourselves from every defilement of body and spirit .
. . (2 Cor. 7:1)

We easily understand the health importance of good food and water, but we seldom consider an even more foundational health ingredient – cleansing. The cleansing and detoxifying process ranks as one of the most important aspects of our physical health. The best food and water, though very important, will have a limited effect apart from a proper understanding of cleansing the body. Let me illustrate:

Suppose you're a dishwasher at a busy restaurant, and the drain on your sink gets plugged up. Your dish water gets dirtier and greasier until you give up and stop washing more dishes. You haven't even gotten the breakfast dishes done when the manager comes in telling you to hurry up because the lunch hour is approaching. When you explain your clogged drain problem, he suggests that you just add more hot water and detergent and keep washing. Now how long do your suppose you can do that before the dishes are not getting clean? Similarly, how long can you sustain your body by just adding more nutrients in without first cleaning out the toxins?

DISEASE THEORIES

In my booklet, *The Sick & Tired Manual*[1], I discuss the three basic theories of illness, of what makes us "sick and tired." Most people have been taught the **germ theory** – the idea that different germs cause different diseases, and therefore you take a germ-killing drug to solve your health problems. This view of course originated with Louis Pasteur in the nineteenth century. While today virtually everyone has signed on to Pasteur's theory, this was not the case during his life, a life filled with critics. Pasteur's most eminent critic was the great French physician and physiologist, the "Father of Experimental Medicine," Claude Bernard, who did not believe germs were the root cause of our health problems. Instead, Bernard argued that the "terrain" was the root cause – the environment you provided in the body for the germs to grow or not grow in. Apparently Dr. Bernard's view eventually got through to Pasteur, who reportedly said on his deathbed:

The germ is nothing; the terrain is everything.

In other words, "Claude Bernard was right – germs are **not** the root cause of disease."

This could be convincingly illustrated a number of ways. For example, suppose we go out to a swamp on a 95 degree August day. As we look at the stagnant water, covered with green slime, infested with bugs, I say to you, "Isn't it amazing the way these bugs made this swamp?" You would think I was crazy making such a ridiculous remark, replying to me, "The bugs didn't make the swamp; the swamp made the bugs." It is that stagnant water that, to use Claude Bernard's terminology, provided a "terrain" for the germs to propagate in. Likewise a free-flowing stream wouldn't provide the terrain and be so infested with bugs. The point is simple: When your body is a stagnant swamp, germs propagate as a *secondary* cause of disease, but when your body is like that free-flowing stream, you stay healthy. However, when you believe the "germ theory," you believe that the bugs make the swamp.

The second disease theory is more common in natural medicine circles – **deficiency theory**. The idea here is that different vitamin and mineral deficiencies are the root cause of our health problems, and taking vitamin and mineral supplements is the answer. Though there's a lot of truth in this view, it runs into three problem questions most people can't answer:

Which nutrients am I deficient in?

Which supplements will actually work in my body?

How much of those supplements, dosage-wise, do I need?

Though many studies have shown widespread nutrient deficiencies in the population, I believe this, like the germ theory, misses the root cause of most of our health problems – **toxicity**. Thus, cleansing and detoxifying the body ranks as a more fundamental step for achieving better health.

SOURCES OF TOXINS

Before talking about cleansing and purifying the body of toxins, let's first examine what toxins are and where they come from. Simply stated a toxin is a poison. Dr. Julian Kenyon in his book, *21st Century Medicine*, lists seven *categories* of "common toxins" typically found in our bodies[2]:

Industrial chemicals

Pesticides

Food additives

Dead bacteria or viruses

Medical drugs

Hydrocarbon-based chemicals

Heavy metals

Let me emphasize that these are just general *categories* of toxins with thousands of possible individual toxins in some of these groups. For example, there are over 10,000 chemical additives approved for use in the American food supply as colorings, flavorings, preservatives, etc. No person's life, even in the most remote areas, is immune from contact with the thousands of chemical solvents, fertilizers, pesticides, cosmetics, drugs, and you name it that daily touch our lives.

But how do we get so toxic? Where do all these toxins come from? In the case of the seven categories above, it's pretty obvious that these toxins are largely the result of modern "civilization." They represent *foreign things taken into the body* from the outside. God did not design our bodies to handle these "man made" poisons. Thus our bodies are stuck trying to either (1) get rid of the toxins, or if they can't do that, (2) store the toxins.

DENTAL MERCURY TOXICITY

Though we ingest toxins daily from refined, chemical-laden foods, impure chemical-laden water, plus a wide variety of environmental chemical exposures, one of the most interesting, though highly controversial, toxin sources is from mercury amalgam dental fillings. Most of the 100 million Americans with amalgam dental fillings are unaware their fillings contain the highly toxic heavy metal, mercury, since they are more commonly called by the misnomer "silver dental fillings," in spite of the fact that they are only 30% silver, but 50% mercury.

During most of the 150 year usage of mercury amalgam dental fillings, the conventional dental establishment has maintained that once the mercury was mixed with the other metals and hardened into the tooth, the mercury didn't escape. However, today's high tech analytical methods like scanning electron microscopy and mercury vapor analyzers have shown that mercury most definitely *does* leak out of the fillings. For example, research done in Sweden by corrosion chemist, Dr. Jaro Pleva, found that a five-year-old mercury filling that was originally 50% mercury then had only 27% mercury[3]. So what happened to the other 23%? It escaped into your body.

It is ironic: The Environmental Protection Agency regards dental mercury as a toxic substance in the dentist's office both *before* it is put into a patient's mouth and *after* it is removed from a patient's mouth. It is a tightly regulated toxic substance with significant fines for mishandling. Are we really supposed to believe that the *only* place mercury amalgam is non-toxic is inside someone's mouth?

Keep in perspective that mercury dental amalgam is just one example of tens of thousands of possible toxins which may affect your body. Take the potential hazard of mercury amalgam and multiply it by the legions of toxins threatening us, and you begin to get the picture of what a significant problem toxicity is. But taking toxins into the body from the *outside* is only part of the problem. There's another even more interesting and problematic method of getting toxic.

SELF-PRODUCED TOXINS

As vile as the toxins taken in from outside the body are, they pale in significance to the toxins you make *inside* your body. *Self-produced* toxins results from poor digestion and poor elimination resulting in putrefaction. My Number One Rule of Health is simply this:

> **Anything that you eat that you don't properly digest, assimilate, and eliminate becomes a toxin.**

Even the "best," "organically grown," "natural" healthy food can produce toxicity courtesy of a poorly functioning digestive tract. J. H. Tilden, MD, early in the 20th century wrote and lectured widely on the subject of self-produced toxicity, saying in one of his books:

> *. . . the human body can be poisoned from pure, wholesome food, as well as from impure food, and the mind, as well as the body, may cause inoxious foods and secretions to become noxious.*[4]

COMPROMISED DIGESTION

We have two basic aspects of digestion, which in turn may lead to this self-produced toxicity Dr. Tilden wrote about, summarized in a first question of:

How digestible is my food?

Much of the food people eat today is not especially digestible, particularly the additive –laden "junk food" that neither spoils on the shelf nor breaks down in your digestive tract. I call this phenomenon **embalming the living**.

But indigestibility of food is not just a matter of chemical preservatives, since certain foods, like meats, are just more difficult to digest. Though a normal digestive system can handle limited amounts of meat fine, most Americans eat large amounts of meat two or three times per day – a habit not compatible with the capacity of our digestive systems. Likewise, improper combining of different types of food (fruits, starches, proteins) may thwart the digestibility of a given food.

After asking how digestible our food is, we must then ask the second question:

How good is my digestion?

Digestion is a function of adequate secretions of various digestive factors such as hydrochloric acid and pepsin in the stomach and different pancreatic enzymes in the small intestine. Overeating, especially of animal proteins, again may so overwhelm the digestive capacity that these secretions diminish. For example, many health authorities state that most people of age 40 have inadequate hydrochloric acid secretions. Other digestive secretions may similarly be exhausted. The end result is the same – incomplete digestion and assimilation leading to toxic putrefaction.

POOR ELIMINATION

Yet digestion is only the first part of the problem leading to toxicity, as said in my Number One Rule of Health:

> *Anything that you don't properly digest, assimilate and eliminate becomes a toxin.*

Suppose you take a piece of raw steak out of the refrigerator, put it on a platter and leave it on the kitchen window sill for three days during 95 degree summer heat. What happens? Putrefaction. What if you take the same piece of meat and put it in your digestive tract for three days, not at 95 degrees or 98.6, but at the colon temperature of 104 degrees. Do you still get putrefaction? You bet!

More than any other aspect of digestion, poor elimination leads to self-produced toxicity. We're talking about the glorious subject of constipation! Few people realize how much of a problem this is. One cancer authority told me early in my career that the average cancer patient had one bowel movement every eight days! In my clinics our staff frequently sees people having one bowel movement every three days, just as with my steak on the window sill illustration. A significant number have only one bowel movement every week, and I've even seen clients having as little as one elimination every *three weeks!*

Ironically, most constipated people don't think it's that big a problem. Do you know why? I believe it's mainly the result of misinformation from the conventional medical profession, especially as found in medical advisor books and newspaper medical question and answer columns, in that whenever the subject of constipation comes up, the stock answer is:

> *"Normal is whatever is normal for you."*

Now is that insane or what? Can you believe that someone actually goes to college and medical school to come up with such nonsensical advice as, "Normal is whatever is normal for you?"

Mere common sense would dictate that there should be some correlation between "intake" and "elimination" as it relates to the digestive process. Studies of primitive peoples who eat more natural foods and are physically active find that they generally have a bowel movement to correspond with each meal they eat. Thus, "normal" for most of us should be two or even three bowel movements per day, though some people might retain good health with just one per day. However, anything less than one bowel movement per day is definitely abnormal and unhealthy, inviting putrefaction and resultant toxicity.

CAUSES OF CONSTIPATION

There are physical causes of constipation, but there are also *non-physical* causes. The three main physical causes are simply:

Lack of fiber in the diet

Lack of pure water in the diet

Lack of exercise

I think most people have been adequately bombarded with thousands of commercials on fiber in the diet, so I won't belabor this self-evident point, but what about pure water. As discussed earlier in my chapter on water, we need both the right *quality* and *quantity* of water for optimum health. The general rule of thumb is to divide your body weight in pounds in two and drink that number of ounces of water daily, an amount that typically far exceeds the average person's consumption. Inactivity slows everything down in the body, including the bowels, while exercise stimulates the normal bowel action.

The *non-physical* cause of constipation is:

Deposition of emotional stress

Because our bodies weren't created to handle emotional stress (it being a result of the Fall), they really don't know what to do with the stress we take in. It often ends up simply *deposited* in an organ or muscle. The digestive tract in general is the favorite repository for our emotional stress, particularly the colon. One doctor quoted in the classic work on emotional stress and health, *How to Live 365 Days a Year*, by John Schindler, M.D., stated it this way;

> *The colon is the mirror of the mind. When the mind gets tight, the colon gets tight.*[5]

And when the colon gets tight, what do you think we're talking about? Constipation and the resulting toxicity. In a subsequent chapter we'll look at emotional stress in more detail and how to win over it. Our next question, though, is how does the body respond to toxicity?

RESPONSE TO TOXINS

In a nutshell, the body's response to toxins, whether those from the outside or self-produced toxins is to either:

Get rid of them (body's preferred method)

Store them (if it can't get rid of them)

Make no mistake, your body is always detoxifying through the bowel, lungs, liver, skin and so on. The question is whether those organs of detoxification can handle the load you're laying on them. Most people have utterly overwhelmed their body's detoxifying capacity through:

Eating the modern American junk food diet

Taking in thousands of environmental toxins

Having inefficient digestion

Living a high stress life

In addition to these factors, most people "roadblock" the body's *automatic* detoxifying process rather than help it along. This phenomenon is best explained by the Theory of Homotoxicology (study of toxins in man) by the late Hans-Heinrich Reckeweg, M.D. of Germany.

THEORY OF HOMOTOXICOLOGY

Dr. Reckeweg taught that *illness is merely an expression of the body's healing process* in response to "homotoxins," that is, "man poisons." He described six possible "phases" the body can go through in its attempt to get rid of the toxins we take in or self-produce. His first three phases are *humoral*, that is, located in the fluids of the body outside the cells such as the blood or lymph. His second three phases are *cellular*, that is, located inside the cell. The first three phases involve detoxification and excretion of homotoxins, while the second three involve cell damage by the homotoxins which the body is trying to repair. Specifically they are:[6]

Excretion Phase – Body attempts to get rid of toxins via the feces, urine, catarrh, menstrual bleeding, discharges from infected wounds, etc.

Reaction Phase – Inflammatory reactions develop such as eczema, enteritis, pharyngitis, tonsillitis, appendicitis, etc.

Deposition Phase – More or less permanent cellular change due to toxin deposition with resulting conditions such as gout, benign tumors, cysts, rheumatism, etc.

Impregnation – Toxins are now present inside the cell such as with liver damage (cirrhosis), lung diseases (asbestos toxicity), etc.

Degeneration Phase – Cellular degeneration due to long-term presence of toxins in the cells resulting in osteoarthritis, emphysema, heart attacks, etc.

Neo-Plastic Phase – Development of cancer in cells affected by toxins.

DEALING WITH TOXICITY

Where your body goes in this progression of homotoxicology's six phases depends upon which of two basic responses you choose to follow with your illness and its underlying toxicity:

Suppress the Symptom

Eliminate the Cause

Most often "suppressing the symptoms" is done by taking some kind of drug whose pharmacology relates only to the disease symptoms, not the underlying causes.

For example, someone takes an aspirin for a headache. The aspirin merely deadens the sensitivity of the body to the headache rather than in any way relating to the underlying cause. *We don't get headaches because our bodies are deficient in aspirin!* The cause of the headache could be constipation, food sensitivity, not drinking enough water, spinal misalignment, emotional stress or other possibilities. Bottom line is simply this: Suppressing the symptoms does not address the underlying toxicity that is the root cause of the problem. The key point is this in Reckeweg's theory: When you suppress the symptom, the toxin remains and is driven to a deeper phase for the body to deal with it. Thus, people move from the initial excretion phase all the way down to the cancerous phase.

However, when we choose to *eliminate the cause*, the direction reverses. Instead of going to the deeper homotoxicology phases, the process turns around leading back to health. We eliminate the cause simply by letting the body detoxify and helping it do that more easily.

Let me share a very practical illustration of how "suppressing the symptoms" versus "eliminating the cause" works. Suppose you're a young mother with a baby who has diarrhea. After a couple of days of this you become concerned enough to go to your pediatrician, who immediately diagnoses, "Your baby has diarrhea," which you already knew, and then scratches out a prescription for an anti-diarrhea drug. Sure enough, within a few hours the diarrhea's gone – another triumph for modern medicine, or is it? Dr. Reckeweg would say that the diarrhea was simply the body's *excretion phase* trying to get rid of the toxin. The drug *suppressed* the toxin, merely driving it to a deeper level for the body to deal with the next time.

"Next time" comes a few months later when your baby develops a skin rash you can't get rid of. This time you go to the dermatologist, who writes out another prescription, probably for a corticosteroid ointment that you rub on. The skin rash dutifully goes away making everyone happy again . . . everyone *except* the baby's body that has again had its toxicity suppressed rather than eliminated! We're now down to the second phase, the *reaction phase*, with the toxin still there and now forced to go even deeper.

The next manifestation of this suppressed toxin comes some time later with a recurrent ear infection, for which you now go to the ear, nose and throat doctor. This practitioner prescribes a course of antibiotics, which clears up the infection in a couple of days, but also moves the toxin deeper, creating the third phase of *deposition*.

Now somewhere during this disgusting process the body basically gets fed up, in effect saying:

> *I'm tired of trying to get rid of these toxins. I tried to get rid of them through the bowel with the diarrhea – they wouldn't let me do that. Then I tried to get rid of them through the skin – they wouldn't let me do that. Then I tried to eliminate the toxins through the lymphatic areas in the head – they wouldn't let me do that. I'm going to quit trying to get rid of these toxins and just go rent a toxin warehouse and store this stuff.*

And that is exactly what often happens – the body "rents" a toxin warehouse which sometimes we call a tumor. Then Mom, when you feel that lump on your baby, you're really scared and run off to the surgeon. After the body has walled off the toxins in the tumor (since you wouldn't let it get rid of those toxins at the excretion, reaction or deposition levels), your well-intentioned surgeon goes in and cuts the whole thing open releasing the toxins again.

At virtually every step we do just the opposite of what would detoxify and heal the body. We tend to compete with the body's natural detoxifying process instead of complement it. The key to health is to stop suppressing symptoms and start eliminating toxic causes of disease. Let's look at a specific Toxin Elimination Program.

TOXIN ELIMINATION

We've discussed how toxins become a root health problem for us, but how do we get rid of them? Let me share a Five-Step Toxin Elimination Program:

Step One – Stop Toxic Input

Maybe it would be more realistic to say, "Reduce toxic input," since it's impossible to totally eliminate taking *any* toxins into your body. Nevertheless, since you control over 90 percent of your toxic input, you are the key to reducing it.

Begin with getting off junk food. Nutrient refined, additive-laden foods are probably the number one source of not only external toxins, but the self-produced toxins as well, since they adversely affect your digestive tract function. My booklet, *The Junk Food Withdrawal Manual*, tells you how to easily make dietary changes to more natural foods in a simple twelve week program.

Second, get off of "junk water," that is, tap water. As discussed in the previous chapter, the typical municipal water supply is a chemical feast you don't want to partake in. I suggest drinking only distilled water, though almost any filtering method will be some improvement over tap water.

Third, avoid drugs. Because drugs are generally synthetic substances, they are treated by the body as a toxin. While there are instances in which drugs must be used to save or sustain life, you don't have to take an aspirin or a cold medication or a sinus antibiotic every time you have the slightest symptoms. Remember that the drugs only cover the symptom, instead of resolving the underlying cause, and thus just add more toxicity to the body. Make drugs the last resort instead of the first resort they have become for the average person.

Fourth, reduce chemical toxicities from soaps, shampoos and cosmetics. Understand that some of whatever you put on the outside of your body is absorbed in. Especially avoid anti-perspirant soaps and deodorants, which normally contain highly toxic aluminum compounds. Dandruff shampoos are likewise highly toxic, not to mention that dandruff usually responds to some basic nutritional supplementation. Most cosmetics contain very objectionable ingredients that again add to the body's toxic input. More natural ingredient soaps, shampoos and cosmetics are available at most health food stores.

Step Two – Detoxifying Fasts and Diets

Offering many different options, detoxifying fasts and diets accentuate the cleansing process in the body. Different health problems and individual constitutions will dictate the best method, the most basic being simply a plain, distilled water fast for one to three days. Although this is an excellent general cleansing method for most people, some will prefer or respond better to juice fasting. Those prone to low blood sugar may do better with the juices to help keep their blood sugar levels up.

In my booklet, *The Sick & Tired Manual*, I describe an Eleven Day Elimination Diet, which combines juice fasting with eventually eating whole fruits and vegetables. This type of cleansing approach, which may be abbreviated to seven days, can be the most popular, in that it allows you eat all you want of the particular foods used.

Step Three – Colon Cleansing

Having discussed earlier the problem of colon toxicity, its seems logical to implement a special cleansing program for this vital organ. Again, there are several possible options:

The most basic approach is using a psyllium husk powder shaken into juice or water. Psyllium swells up in liquid providing a bulking supplement to cleanse the colon. Unlike other fibers such as wheat bran, psyllium is gentler and less irritating to the intestinal walls, though very effective. Flaxseed powder, fruit pectin and other fibers are also possibilities in this category.

Second, herbal laxatives may be used when bowels are irregular. Unlike drug laxatives, herbal laxatives do not have the harsh, habit-forming characteristics and thus can be used more safely. If someone is very constipated and perhaps has a history of chronic constipation, *both* psyllium *and* herbal laxatives may need to be used together.

Third, we have enemas, a bowel detoxification approach once a common method used by both mothers and doctors, though unfamiliar today to most. When I tell a mother to give her child an enema, she usually looks at me like I just suggested some method of medieval torture! Cleansing the colon directly with an enema simply helps it get rid of toxins faster. Enemas can be helpful most anytime you're sick, as well as to enhance detoxification during a cleansing diet or fast. Some suggestions:

Obtain a plastic enema bucket (open at the top), if possible. The water flow in easier than with hot water bottle enema syringes that are more common.

Lie on your left side on a towel on the bathroom floor with the enema bucket sitting on the closed toilet seat lid. If the enema bucket is too high it will produce too much water pressure and resulting discomfort.

Use 16 – 32 oz. of distilled water. In some cases lemon juice, liquid chlorophyll or herbs are appropriate to add to the enema water.

Relax and breathe deeply as the water flows in. Massaging the abdomen may help water inflow.

Holding a piece of toilet tissue against the anus tends to take away the urge to expel, but don't overdo it. Expel into the toilet before getting too uncomfortable.

Taking a second enema immediately after the first is usually helpful, since there is less pressure to eliminate.

Fourth, we have colonic irrigations, basically a "high tech" enema done with a machine by a trained therapist who controls the inflow or water and outflow of waste through switching a valve. Utilizing a clear section on the exit tube, the therapist can see what kinds of deposits are being removed from the colon. By varying water temperatures and doing abdominal massage and other techniques, a very thorough cleansing of the colon can be executed. Though some people recommend colonics for most anyone, I usually reserve this approach for those with more chronic colon problems.

Step Four – Vitamin-Mineral-Herbal Supplementation

Several vitamins and mineral have special detoxifying properties that are helpful. Vitamins A and C are probably the most basic for cleansing the lymph, liver and blood, as well as stimulating the immune system. Nutrient minerals such as calcium and magnesium are key in *displacing* toxic minerals like the heavy metals. Herbs provide yet another detoxification possibility – milk thistle, red clover and many others may be appropriate, according to individual testing.

Step Five -- Homeopathic Remedies

Homeopathic detoxifying remedies consist of micro-dilutions of whatever toxins we're trying to get rid of. While the toxin itself produces ill effects, the homeopathic dilution of the toxin has the opposite effect, a neutralizing and detoxifying effect, stimulating the body to eliminate that toxin. The homeopathic remedy is akin to hanging up a "wanted poster," alerting the body's "police force" to apprehend and get rid of the toxic "criminal." Another type of homeopathic supplement, called a "drainage formula," helps this detoxifying process along by stimulating the elimination pathways such as the bowel, liver, kidneys, skin, etc. This type of supplementation program requires specific testing for compatibility, as we do in our nutritional clinics.

CONCLUSION

Proper detoxification is foundational to our physical health. God created your body to detoxify -- and it will if you'll only let it rather than getting in the way. Years of symptom suppression can in most cases still be reversed with the help of proper eating and supplementation. But there's an additional healing and detoxifying method we'll cover next.

Chapter 4

By the Sweat of Your Brow

If anyone is not willing to work . . . (II Thessalonians 3:10a)

Is "exercise" essential for good health, or is there something better – something more biblical? Actually the Bible has nothing to say about "exercise," but quite a lot to say about "work." God has a special design in physical work that we will profit from discovering.

"Exercise" is just a type of work, really a "counterfeit work," invented by modern people who no longer have to physically work for their living. Interestingly enough, the healthiest peoples in the world don't have aerobic dance, jogging, health spas, and the like, *but they all have physical work.* Let's look at the scriptural basis of work and how it ties in with your total person health.

WORK IN THE GARDEN

> *The Lord God took the man and put him in the Garden of Eden to work it and keep it.* (Genesis 2:15)

God designed man to work, to be productive, to be useful, and not to just sit around. Note that this passage is *before* the Fall. Man was working even in the perfect, sinless Eden. I think we can therefore assume that we will also have work to do in the New Heaven and Earth of eternity – none of this lying around on a cloud plucking a harp nonsense!

Doing meaningful work, including at least some physical work, stands as a primary ingredient of a fulfilling life. People who work hard physically seldom get sick – they're also a lot more emotionally stable, not having the time or energy to be neurotic! I personally believe this is one of the main reasons that traditional hard-working, profusely sweating farmers have been such a stable part of our population. But how that all changed when farming became more like any other business with the farmer being more of a business manager than a laborer, when air-conditioned combines that you could operate wearing a business suit replaced hot, uncomfortable tractors (not to mention horses before that).

What happens when people cease from doing meaningful work? A psychologist once told me that the average lifespan after retirement for those *not* continuing in some kind of meaningful work is *two years*. I have often asked people in my seminars what the leading cause of death is in the United States. I would get replies like "heart disease," "cancer," and the like – to all of which I would say, "incorrect." Actually I believe the leading cause of death is the Social Security system. What does it do? It encourages people to stop working, usually well before physical limitations would so dictate. It has instilled in the mindset of our culture the concept of "retirement," a concept utterly foreign to the Scripture, and therefore a concept that brings death. In Psalm 92:14 we read of the godly person:

> *They will still bear fruit in old age; they are ever full of sap and green.*

You don't get "fruit" without cultivation and without work, do you?

THE BLESSING OF THE CURSE

Although the Fall of Man brought a curse, that curse actually contains a blessing as related to work:

> *Cursed is the ground because of you; in pain you shall eat of it all the days of your life; thorns and thistles it shall bring forth for you; and you shall eat the plants of the field. By the sweat of your face you shall eat bread, till you return to the*

ground, for out of it you were taken; for you are dust, and to dust you shall return. (Genesis 3:17-19)

After the Fall survival depended on growing food to survive. Man went from the tending of a garden to the toil of farming. The curse we all have inherited from Adam requires physical labor for us to survive. That's the "curse" part, but there's also a blessing hidden within that curse – physical work is a key ingredient of life, health, and survival. It feels good to sweat. It's healthy because it fulfills God's command to the first man.

Is it any wonder that executives and others with vocations that do not involve physical labor have such a problem with heart attacks and other maladies? Though, as a nutritionist, I hate to admit it, physically hard working people can eat a lousy diet and often be healthier than people eating an excellent diet who do not physically work. God is not mocked – His covenant with Adam stands, no matter how many "labor-saving" devices we invent. A beautiful verse summarizes the fulfillment and peace of hard physical work this way:

> *The sleep of the working man is pleasant, whether he eats little or much.* (Ecclesiastes 5:12a)

THE GLORY OF LABOR

Although work has been inseparably tied to health and survival since the Fall, socialistic government structures keep trying to change that design – to make it possible to live without working. Perhaps the greatest tragedy of our growing welfare state, beyond its financial injustice to the productive, is its utter destruction of the emotional and physical health of its recipients. The "dole" decimates self-esteem, while being given the opportunity to work in even the most menial job, is satisfying and fulfilling.

God's idea is that we work so as not to be in need, to be able to help others in need, and to stay out of trouble bred by idleness. Let's look at some scriptures:

Let the thief no longer steal, but rather let him labor, doing honest work with his own hands, so that he may have something to share with anyone in need. (Ephesians 4:28)

. . . aspire to live quietly, and to mind your own affairs, and to work with your hands, as we instructed you, so that you may live properly before outsiders and be dependent on no one. (I Thessalonians 4:11-12)

For even when we were with you, we would give you this command: If anyone is not willing to work, let him not eat. For we hear that some among you walk in idleness, not busy at work, but busybodies. Now such persons we command and encourage in the Lord Jesus Christ to do their work quietly and to earn their own living. (II Thessalonians 3:10-12)

Work is glorious to God, beautiful in His plan of redeeming mankind from the Fall. Work is practical in meeting our needs and the needs of others, not to mention preventing us from engaging in sins of idleness.

EXERCISE VS. WORK

The great problem today is simply that most of us, myself included, earn our living *without* performing physical labor. Instead of the "sweat of our brow," we put bread on the table with the sweat of our brains. While that "brain labor" fulfills at least part of God's purpose – not being in need – what about His other purposes? What about the physical health benefits of physical labor? It just doesn't happen with today's mostly non-physical work force. Is it any wonder that "desk jobs" are notorious for their promotion of heart disease, obesity, and a host of other epidemic health problems?

So is "exercise" the answer? Or is physical work the answer? Being a great proponent of physical exercise, it's hard for me to admit it, but I doubt that "exercise" would really be needed if we did proper physical work. The world's healthiest people have never heard of aerobics, of running to no place in particular, or exercise machines, or lifting weights for no real reason. Instead they just work and work hard at what they do.

The Scripture is void of any concept of what we call "exercise." So where did it come from, then? Like many of our other humanistic concepts, we have the ancient Greeks to thank. That, of course, was where the Olympic Games were founded. In the games, as well as in their art and sculpture, the Greeks glorified not God the Creator, but the physical body of man, the creature, fulfilling the very essence of humanism – the glorification of man.

Since I brought up the Olympics, let me add another observation from the modern games, which I used to watch extensively. While I am always amazed at the feats the athletes perform, I also feel a great sadness in the realization of how incredibly hard they work for one moment of fleeting glory, for a medal of no lasting significance. In pondering these feelings I recalled Paul's very similar thoughts on the ancient games:

> *Do you not know that in a race all the runners compete, but only one receives the prize? So run that you may obtain it. Every athlete exercises self-control in all things. They do it to receive a perishable wreath, but we an imperishable. So I do not run aimlessly; I do not box as one beating the air. But I discipline my body and keep it under control, lest after preaching to others I myself should be disqualified.* (I Corinthians 9:24-27)

Don't get me wrong, as I am not saying that exercise or desire to improve your physical body is sinful. But I think the philosophy of "exercise," as practiced in our culture, lacks biblical basis and is therefore optional at best. On the other hand, work, from a biblical point-of-view is hardly optional, but rather is mandatory. Work has a balancing effect on the total person; exercise does not.

Many have made a "religion" out of jogging or bicycling or marathons or whatever (which proves the imbalancing effect to the total person). Some exercise faddists are literally addicted to their exercise. Studies have shown that over-fatiguing the body actually produces LSD-like chemicals. This is yet another example of the "God provides, man perverts" dichotomy. Who would ever think that something as pure and wholesome as running could be turned into a "psychedelic experience?" God provided the body to do work, but we have often perverted work into mere exercise.

Exercise really has no useful end, no objective other than some type of self-glorification. Work, however, has an objective and resulting fulfillment, both psychologically and spiritually, in addition to its physical health benefit.

EXERCISE LESS – WORK MORE

My Dad always found it ironic that taxpayers are forced to fund millions of dollars to build school gymnasiums, swimming pools, and athletic fields, while simultaneously funding buses so kids won't have to walk to school. Children and adults alike ride to a place in order to "exercise." Doesn't that seem a little odd? We often laugh at the tales of previous generations about how many miles they walked to school through the snow in 20 below zero weather, but actually a lot of them did, though perhaps minus some of the exaggeration. It's a given that they were healthier than the average kid today with all the gyms, swimming pools, and P.E. programs.

So what are some practical steps we can implement to get more involved in "work" *so that* we don't have to just settle for the inferior substitute of "exercise?"

1. Walk, Don't Ride – What an enemy of health the automobile has become! It's not just through accidents, but rather in preventing us from walking to fulfill normal obligations. I find it very ironic that most people will get in their car and drive to someplace *in order to exercise*. They drive to a place to go walking, jogging, bicycling or to a health club to work out. Have you ever really thought about how crazy that is? If we used our cars less, we wouldn't have as great a need to exercise.

I once had a friend that who always drove to a health club six or seven blocks from his office. He always drives there – never walks. But if he walked to the health club, he'd probably need less time at the club. But someone says, "Oh, but I don't have time to walk." Really? But you have time to go work out at a health club. Who's kidding whom?

I remember another time when a friend and I were going to lunch at a place in sight, perhaps a quarter of a mile across a shopping center parking lot. It was a beautiful, sunny day, so I said, "Let's walk over." He said, "No, I don't want to walk; that takes too long." Well, by the time you get through the traffic and park the car, walking might take what, one or two minutes longer? Beyond that it would stimulate the appetite, reduce tension (something city driving definitely won't do), and otherwise allow you to step back and enjoy life for a moment, stopping to smell the roses.

Why not look for the opportunities you have to walk? One time I took my car into a garage for some work, and rather than get a ride back to my office, I just walked. It was a mile at most, part of which went through a nice park. It took ten minutes or so and was practical, enjoyable exercise. Another time, in another city, I took my car to the dealer for work and brought my bicycle with me. I rode it four or five miles back to my home and had a great time. Another time I would split wood in the morning before our family Bible study time. Believe me, it was much more satisfying than my morning "exercise" routine.

I have many other examples. After my bout with cancer in 1974, I would walk from our Southern California home on the edge of the city up to our ministry headquarters 1000 feet above the city via a number of back roads. It took about 45 minutes, but it was very therapeutic as a workout, plus giving me time to pray and memorize Scripture. The hundreds of fellow staff members that drove onto the grounds every morning missed so much that I enjoyed.

Another example, instead of involving cars, involves stairs. I make it a habit in moderate sized buildings to use the stairways rather than the elevators. Walking up two or three flights of stairs actually feels pretty good. However, sometimes your intentions can be foiled. I remember many years ago deciding to use the stairs on a 20+ story office building on Wilshire Boulevard in Los Angeles, only to get dead-ended at the fourth floor and having to switch to the elevator. Of course using the stairs for two or three flights usually presents no problem, plus you'll probably get to where you're going faster than you would on the elevator!

If you're really in such a hurry that you can't walk instead of ride or can't climb the stairs instead of taking the elevator, my counsel is simple: Change. Slow down. Stop and smell the roses before your mourners are smelling the roses over your remains.

2. Select Meaningful Activities for Yourself Involving Physical Work – Many examples come to mind, such as yard work. Why pay someone else to do it if you're in desperate need of physical activity? There's also a special emotional and spiritual value with doing such physical labor in or around your own home, a value you won't get working out at your health club. Along the same lines you have all kinds of household work – cleaning, painting, splitting wood, repairing, and the like. Some of these might not require great exertion, but they are nevertheless meaningful physical work.

Of all the possible physical work I personally feel that none is better than gardening, working with the soil to produce food. This activity literally fulfills the command of the Adamic Covenant. There is such an incredible balancing effect that comes from growing food, an effect I believe is due to the fulfillment of God's command to Adam. I think everyone should have some kind of garden and grow at least some of their own food. Beyond just the Adamic Covenant, the health and nutrition benefits of doing this are incredible. God knew that it would be best for us to grow our own food long before the devitalizing effects of commercial agriculture and food distribution had come on the scene.

People who are very involved in gardening have a special peace about them usually. A famous line by George Gurney of the Gurney Seed Company I remember so well was, "I never knew a gardener who needed a psychiatrist." The people who rush everywhere, who drive to their health clubs to work out but haven't the time to walk a few blocks, and who are plagued by the "tyranny of the urgent" usually aren't gardeners.

My point is simply to find some meaningful physical work that really needs to be done. Then you either won't need or will need less "exercise."

WORKING SIX DAYS

God created us with a special balance between the need for work and the need for rest, summarized in the principle of the Sabbath:

> *Remember the Sabbath day, to keep it holy. Six days you shall labor and do all your work, but the seventh day is a Sabbath of the Lord your God; in it you shall not do any work, you or your son or your daughter, your male or your female servant or your cattle or your sojourner who stays with you.* (Exodus 20:8-10)

Though not very popular with present day preachers, the subject of not working on the Sabbath has been preached to death over the centuries. I firmly believe that the "one in seven" resting principle is basic to God's creation of the universe, and therefore, we are most wise to line up with it. However the emphasis on resting on the Sabbath has overshadowed the first part of the command: We first need to work six days before we're entitled to rest one day. The problem with many today is not that they work on the seventh day so much as it is that they don't work on the six days – at least not physically work. When one physically works six days, no persuasive sermons are usually needed about resting on the seventh day.

LEISURE

Does the biblical emphasis on work mean that leisure is bad? Well, let me put it this way – the concept of leisure as promoted in our culture is pretty foreign to the Bible. It too is a concept of Greek philosophy. "Leisure" is defined as "freedom from occupation." The popular idea today is that leisure is the goal of life – make your fortune quickly so you can lie around on the beach in Hawaii the rest of your life. If there's ever been a vain imagination about the ideal life, this has got to be it. Most people who have tried "leisure" find it gets pretty boring after about 30 minutes! "Leisure" as a basic life goal runs counter to God's revealed design for man. It denies the fact that God put us here for a purpose of doing something other than just sitting around watching the scenery.

The emphasis in the Bible is not on "leisure" but rather on "rest," and there is a huge difference. Rest is the necessary ceasing from labor, the fulfillment of the pattern God made for all of the Creation. Rest must be preceded by labor – by work. Rest is defined in the dictionary as:

> *1. A state of quiet or repose*
>
> *2. Freedom from care; peace; quiet*
>
> *3. Sleep*

There are many biblical examples of rest, the Sabbath being perhaps the best. After limiting himself as an example to working six days and resting on the seventh God required the same pattern for man, for the animals man worked, for the land, for indebtedness, and so on. This cycle of work and rest is built into all the creation, and the effects are felt when we violate it.

One of the most beautiful examples of God's provision of rest is found in the life of Elijah. After prophesying the three year drought about to come on the land, God sent him away for some R and R:

> *Go away from here and turn eastward, and hide yourself by the brook of Cherith, which is east of the Jordan. And the ravens brought him bread and meat in the morning and bread and meat in the evening, and he would drink from the brook.* (I Kings 17:3,6)

There is a time in which God's Word to us likewise is, "Go, hide yourself." Times for rest, repose, reflection, recreation (that is "re-creation") are fundamental to our total health in body, mind and spirit. (Note: This topic is more extensively discussed in my book on Christian Personal Retreats – *Face to Face: Meeting God in the Quiet Places* – which is linked at the end of this book.)

CONCLUSION

We live in a culture that has moved a long ways from the biblical design of work in God's overall plan. Humanistic Greek concepts of leisure and exercise for solely the glorification of the body abound. Christians have a grand opportunity to look to the Word of God rather than the prevailing culture for their lifestyle models.

Modern culture has robbed us of the benefits of having to physically work in order to survive. While we cannot deny the reality of modern technology and a culture which requires mental rather than physical sweat to earn a living for most of us, we cannot fully abandon the requirement of physical work, at least if we want to experience the fullness of life and health God intended. Those whose living is made with physical work should rejoice in it, understanding and appreciating the provision of God it represents. Those whose vocation is non-physical in its labor, need to incorporate physical work into their life at home, preferably starting with tilling the land and growing some food as Adam did.

While "exercise" cannot be condemned or rejected, it nevertheless must be regarded as second-best to proper labor. Much of your exercise need can be eliminated simply by re-orienting habits of walking, of doing labor yourself rather than hiring it, and other practical measures. Discovering work and rest in their biblical roles can be a great shot in the arm to your total health in body, mind and spirit.

Chapter 5

Let the Sun Shine

Light is sweet, and it is pleasant for the eyes to see the sun.

(Ecclesiastes 11:7)

"Forty-one degrees. It's forty-one degrees and overcast again." I repeated this familiar refrain many a winter morning during the seventeen winters I spent in the Seattle area, where the sun (especially in winter) is pretty much regarded as an Unidentified Flying Object. With only 164 clear or partly cloudy days per year you can understand why. But what did cloudy, damp weather have to do with health? I found out the hard way.

After developing an adrenal gland failure called Addison's Disease (unrelated to sunshine as far as I know), I developed osteoporosis from corticosteroids required to treat the condition. My bone density didn't really improve much in spite of the comprehensive nutritional supplement program I designed for myself. Prescription drugs, which I later reluctantly accepted, weren't much help either.

Then I started spending winters in Tucson, Arizona with over 300 days of sunshine per year. I absolutely delighted in day after day after day of warm sunshine. I started feeling lots better mood-wise, too. Eventually tests revealed that my osteoporosis was improving. During this same time I moved from Seattle to the high desert of Central Oregon with 263 sunny or mostly sunny days per year. Then I was spending both winter and summer in a drier, sunnier climate. My health continued to improve. My bone density continued to improve. Since moving into the sunshine, I've enjoyed the best health of my life.

AN EPIDEMIC OF "HELIOPHOBIA"

During my winters in a retirement community in Arizona I observed countless little old ladies covered from head to toe making sure not a single ray of sun touched their skin. To this day I can picture their pasty white complexion giving that "death warmed over" look. Ironically, I'm sure they thought they were doing something healthy by avoiding **all** sun exposure.

Let's back up a bit. The sun is the source of all life on this planet. Without it we're all dead. So where did we come up with the brilliant conclusion that the sun was the great enemy of health? In a word – propaganda. Propaganda from doctors, from the government, and from various "health" authorities – all brought to you by their willing lapdogs in the media. They've all given us **heliophobia** – fear of the sun. According to the Environmental Protection Agency (EPA) we should "protect ourselves against ultraviolet light whenever we can see our shadow." Did you get that? The government actually wants you to be **afraid of your shadow**! Spouting that kind of nonsense, I think we had better instead fear the government. Several questions emerge:

Is skin cancer really caused by sunshine?

Is ozone depletion making sunshine more harmful?

Can sunshine prevent disease?

How do we get the right amount of sun exposure?

A WORD FROM OUR CREATOR

God apparently is very big on sunshine. His first act of creation was the creation of light (Genesis 1:3). We read in Genesis 1:16-18:

> *And God made the two great lights – the greater light to rule the day and the lesser light to rule the night – and the stars. And God set them in the expanse of the heavens to give light on the earth, to rule over the day and over the night, and to separate the light from the darkness. And God saw that it was good.*

Did you hear God's commentary? **It was good.** The sun was good. In a world that's constantly telling us the sun is bad, God said, "It was good."

Jesus described the sun as a blessing:

> *For he makes his sun rise on the evil and on the good, and sends rain on the just and on the unjust.* (Matthew 5:45b)

God gives the sun and the rain to all mankind out of his goodness. Theologians refer to this as "common grace." Such a statement presupposes that the sun is in fact good for you. The sheer fact that all life would cease without it should prove the point. In other passages Jesus says the righteous are like the sun:

> *Then the righteous will shine like the sun in the kingdom of their Father.* (Matthew 13:43a)

> *You are the light of the world.* (Matthew 5:14a)

Just as the sun brings life to the physical world, so believers bring light to a spiritually dark and dead world. Let me share one more scripture passage that talks about the sun:

> *For the Lord God is a sun and shield; the Lord bestows favor and honor. No good thing does he withhold from those who walk uprightly.* (Psalm 84:11)

The passage identifies the sun as symbolic of God as he, like the sun, provides light, warmth, protection, energy, and power. Then it says that God, who is a "sun" to us, withholds no good thing. Therefore, by implication the sun is good because God is good.

Biblical passages talking about the sun symbolically are of course not scientific treatises on its benefits. That's not the point. Nevertheless, understanding the exalted references to the sun in scripture should rebuke some of the current paranoia about sun exposure. God's creation, including the sun, is good and **good for us** when properly used.

SKIN CANCER FACTS & FICTION

We are constantly told that sunshine and skin cancer go together. Is sun overexposure really the main cause, though? Scientific research would seem to clearly indicate that ultraviolet (UV) radiation can cause skin cancer. But is it really the primary cause or just a scapegoat for the real causes of this disease? Let's begin by taking a look at the three different kinds of UV light:

1. UVA – UVA is a long wave ultraviolet light most often associated with "black light" that you might see used for entertainment purposes (rock bands in the 60's loved it) or to illuminate fluorescent minerals. Although the sun emits UVA, UVB, and UVC, it's estimated that 99% of the UV radiation that actually reaches the earth's surface is UVA. Medically UVA is used to treat skin conditions such as psoriasis and vitiligo. UVA is regarded as the least harmful, though it can age the skin. Though it penetrates deeply, it generally doesn't cause sunburn, though it can cause premature aging and skin cancer with prolonged exposure. UVA is primarily responsible for the "tanning" effect of the sun. The "tanning process" is actually God's way of protecting us. Darkening the skin by tanning makes the skin less vulnerable to UV radiation.

2. UVB – This medium wave UV only reaches the outer layer of your skin and there has the beneficial effect of producing Vitamin D. It's also the type of radiation that produces sunburn. UVB receives most of the blame by authorities for causing skin cancer, though UVA is increasingly cited as well. Ultraviolet lamps from tanning beds also emit both UVA and UVB.

3. UVC – This short wave UV is the most dangerous, but it is completely blocked by the earth's ozone layer and thus does not affect human, animal or plant life on earth. Artificially produced UVC is primarily known for its germicidal effects.

The basic line we hear is that UV light causes skin cancer, so don't expose yourself to the sun and also use lots of sun block. But how do we explain the fact that people have worked out in the sun for thousands of years without getting skin cancer? How do we explain the fact that the increased incidence of skin cancer is a recent phenomenon occurring at a time when fewer people work outdoors?

OZONE HOLE NONSENSE

The ozone layer around the earth blocks harmful UV radiation, particularly UVC and great majority of the UVB. Many environmentalists push the theory that depletion of the ozone layer by chlorofluorocarbons (CFC's) and other man-caused chemicals accounts for the increase in skin cancer. Part of this theory is the idea that the "ozone hole" – the area over Antarctica that seasonally has the least ozone – is expanding. However, scientists from the German Aerospace Center, after analyzing data from Europe's newest meteorological satellite, say the "ozone hole" is not expanding, but shrinking.

That debate aside, the simple facts show no relationship between the "ozone hole" and increased rates of skin cancer. The largest city near the Antarctic ozone hole is Punta Arenas, Chile. If the environmentalists' theory is correct, we should see higher levels of UV radiation there, along with higher levels of skin cancer. In fact, we observe neither.[2] Conversely, from 1957 to 1984 there was no change in ozone or UV radiation over Norway, but the melanoma rate increased 350% for men and 440% for women.[3] Obviously, we need to find something else, other than UV radiation from ozone depletion, to blame for skin cancer. Let's look at the real causes.

CAUSES OF SKIN CANCER

So if normal sun exposure is not the primary cause of skin cancer, what is? Documented studies point to several other causes:

1. Diet – Most aspects of health ultimately connect to diet, and skin cancer is no exception. University of Minnesota scientists note:

> *Epidemiological and animal-based investigations have indicated that the development of skin cancer is in part associated with poor dietary practices.*[3]

The authors show that while omega 3 fatty acids, as found in fish oils, reduce the risk of skin cancer, omega 6 fatty acids, as found in corn, soy and safflower vegetable oils, increase the risk. The journal *Cancer Research* reported:

Epidemiological, experimental, and mechanistic data implicate omega-6 fat as stimulators and long-chain omega-3 fats as inhibitors of development and progression of a range of human cancers, including melanoma.[4]

The real issue is the ratio between the omega 3 fatty acids, as found in flaxseed and fish oils, and omega 6 fatty acids. The average American today has a 15:1 omega 6 to omega 3 ratio, while it's believed that primitive man had more like a 1:1 ratio. The Japanese have the greatest lifespan of any major nation and have a 3:1 omega 6 to omega 3 ratio. Ratios of 4 to 1 or less correspond with reduced incidence of cardiovascular disease, rheumatoid arthritis and certain types of cancer.

2. Indoor Lighting – Ironically it appears that indoor lighting may be more of a cause of skin cancer than sunlight. Artificial, indoor light is a phenomenon of just the last hundred years. Could this be another reason why our sweaty, sun-drenched forbears were not plagued by skin cancer? A US Navy study found that the most malignant melanoma was found not in people who worked in the sun, but with **people who worked indoors under artificial light!** They found that most of these skin cancers occur on areas of the body not even exposed to the sun.[5]

Another study, published in The Lancet, similarly found that it was not sunlight, but **fluorescent light** that caused more than twice the melanoma risk – another "modern" development. The study actually found that long exposure to full-spectrum sunlight actually "immunized" people from the later development of melanoma.[6] I would hasten to add that if you work indoors, at least install full-spectrum fluorescent lights to approximate the beneficial radiation from the sun. They're not as good as real sunlight, but they're miles ahead of the very unnatural light that comes from standard fluorescent tubes.

The late Dr. John Ott, inventor of time-lapse photography and famous for his work with the health effects of full-spectrum lighting, found that the light from fluorescent tubes (plus TV and computer screens) causes red blood cells to clump together, resulting in reduced alertness, fatigue, and increased heart attack and stroke risk. Ott became interested in full-spectrum light when his arthritis was cured after he fell and broke his glasses! Ott repeatedly saw terminal cancer patients get well simply by taking off their sunglasses and prescription glasses and then getting out in the sun. Jane Wright, M.D., Director of Cancer Research at Bellevue Memorial Medical Center in New York City in 1959 implemented Ott's approach and saw 14 of 15 progressive tumor patients have no growth in their tumors. The one who didn't improve sat outdoors, but still kept his UV blocking prescription glasses on.

3. Sunscreen – What? Sunscreen? Isn't that supposed to prevent skin cancer? Yes and yes, but no it doesn't stop skin cancer. Sunscreen is just another hoax. The basic rule of propaganda is simply to repeat a lie often enough and people will come to believe it as the truth. Sunscreen blocks out the ultraviolet light that can benefit your health in the name of protecting you from skin cancer. It thus prevents Vitamin D production and its profound cancer preventing effects, which we'll discuss later in this chapter.

Another issue with sunscreen is the toxicity of the chemicals used. Anything you put on your skin gets absorbed into your body. For example, most sunscreens contain octyl methoxycinnamate (OMC), which Norwegian scientists found to kill mouse cells even low doses.[6] Some associate the increase in skin cancer with none other than the parallel increase in sunscreen usage, noting that sunscreen chemicals themselves may be carcinogenic, having never been safety tested or safety approved by the FDA.

4. Chlorinated Water – At least two studies and other reports link drinking and/or bathing in chlorinated water with an increase in melanoma.[7, 8] Other studies tie swimming in chlorinated water with increased melanoma risk.[9, 10] Of course, most people today are drinking and bathing in chlorinated water. I recommend drinking distilled water and using a chlorine-removing shower filter to eliminate this hazard. Again we see the difference with our "modern" life as compared to 100 years ago when chlorine intake through the water supply was not nearly as common – and neither was skin cancer.

5. Hormone Replacement Therapy (HRT) – The United States, Australia and Europe are the three primary areas of the world using both birth control and hormone replacement therapy (HRT). Is it then just a coincidence that these same three areas also have the most melanoma? In one study all the women who developed melanoma before age 40 had used birth control pills, resulting in a three times greater risk.[11] Meanwhile, less developed nations, where people are more likely to be outside working in the sun, somehow escape being at the top of the list for skin cancer.

So what's the conclusion? Simply this: Sun exposure is a **secondary** cause in the development of skin cancer. We have to get our eyes off of secondary causes by asking the right questions:

Why should skin cancer be dramatically rising at this time, when if anything, people are spending more time out of the sun?

Why have people managed to work out in the sun for thousands of years not getting skin cancer, while now, all of a sudden, with most people working indoors, skin cancer is a huge health problem?

Apparently, people in the past were not compromised by the primary causes of skin cancer. Normal sun exposure will only produce skin cancer when diet, indoor lighting, sunscreen, chlorine, prescription hormones, or other lifestyle factors compromise the body's resistance.

VITAMIN D DEFICIENCY

The greatest problem created by heliophobia is vitamin D deficiency. William B. Grant, one the world's top vitamin D researchers, states that 80% of all Americans are deficient in this essential vitamin. Needless to say, the sun is the primary source of vitamin D, through the reaction of ultraviolet light with the skin. Is it any surprise that most people are vitamin D deficient after decades of "stay out of the sun" propaganda?

Most northern latitudes don't get enough sun during the fall, winter or spring for adequate vitamin D production. This would include latitudes above 35°— north of Los Angeles, Phoenix, Oklahoma City, Memphis and Raleigh – in other words, about two-thirds of the U. S. Originally people lived in the more tropical areas of the earth and got lots of sunshine. But throughout history, migration to more northerly latitudes has occurred, not to mention the movement from the more sunny country skies to less sunny city dwelling places. Add to that the "help" of health authorities telling you to stay out of the sun and bathe yourself in sunscreen whenever you go outdoors. Is it any wonder we have a vitamin D deficiency problem?

Since most people can't get adequate sun exposure other than during the summer, vitamin D supplementation is usually essential, particularly in the winter. The 400 IU dosage typically found in multi-vitamins isn't nearly enough. Many health practitioners now recommend 2000 – 4000 IU's per day when you cannot get enough sun to turn your skin slightly pink. Some have even proposed an upper limit as high as 10,000 IU's.[12] Since a study in the *American Journal of Clinical Nutrition* found 4000 IU's per/day to be safe, I don't go much beyond that limit with my clients.[13]

"SUNSHINE DEFICIENCY" DISEASES

Could many of our health problems simply be the result of not getting enough sunshine? Health authorities are finding more and more diseases related to vitamin D deficiency – in other words, **sunshine deficiency diseases**:

1. Bone Diseases -- First of all, we think of bone diseases in relationship to vitamin D deficiency – rickets, osteoporosis, osteopenia and osteomalacia. We expect those conditions to result from lack of vitamin D, but surprisingly many other health problems also have a D connection.

2. High Blood Pressure -- Some of the latest findings concern heart disease and high blood pressure. Researchers first observed, beginning in the 1940's, a correlation between high blood pressure and people living in temperate latitudes where there is less sunshine and vitamin D production. A recent study confirmed this, finding a direct correlation between distance one lives from the equator and increases in blood pressure.[14] Closely related to this finding is the fact that blood pressure tends to be higher in the winter with diminished sunshine and the resulting deficiency of vitamin D.

Renin and angiotensin directly affect blood pressure. The enzyme, renin, produces angiotensin I, which is converted to angiotensin II by ACE (angiotensin converting enzyme). Angiotensin II causes a constriction of the blood vessels, thus resulting in higher blood pressure. "ACE inhibitor" drugs lower blood pressure by interfering with the ACE enzyme that produces Angiotensin II. So where does vitamin D fit in? Vitamin D controls the level of renin and angiotensin, thus regulating blood pressure. Many studies show the relationship between vitamin D and blood pressure. One study, reported in the *Lancet*, noted that ultraviolet light lowers blood pressure of those mildly hypertensive.[15] Two other clinical trials found vitamin D to lower both systolic and diastolic blood pressure.[16, 17] Researchers find that the higher your blood levels of vitamin D, the lower your blood pressure.[18, 19]

3. Diabetes – Could vitamin D levels be a factor in diabetes? That's what a couple of studies on pregnant women and their children suggest. The first study reviewed the women's vitamin D intake and then, several years later, monitored the children borne to them for diabetes incidence. The women who supplemented vitamin D during pregnancy produced significantly fewer Type I diabetic children.[20] In conducting a follow-up study on the children, researchers discovered that those given 2000 IU's of vitamin D daily starting at age one had a 80% reduction in diabetes risk.[21]

4. Autoimmune Diseases – If the body's own immune system attacks healthy tissue, we call it an "autoimmune" disease. One of the most common such diseases, Multiple Sclerosis (MS), is the deterioration of the myelin sheaths around the nerves, resulting in various crippling neuromuscular symptoms. Like many other diseases, MS is more common away from the equator in the temperate latitudes. Couple a northerly latitude with often overcast skies and you'll usually find a high incidence of MS. This is exactly the case in Seattle, which has one of the highest rates of the disease of any area in the country.

What of other autoimmune diseases such as rheumatoid arthritis, lupus, sarcoidosis, scleroderma, myasthenia gravis, ankylosing spondylitis, and the like? Might these, as well as MS, be helped by simply getting some sunshine and/or significant vitamin D supplementation?

Other diseases vitamin D deficiency may lead to include inflammatory diseases, infertility, PMS, Chronic Fatigue Syndrome and general muscle pain and weakness. But none of these is the worst health problem.

CANCER & VITAMIN D

Cancer may well be the worst result of our fear of the sun and resulting vitamin D deficiency. A Creighton University School of Medicine study found that increased vitamin D levels could reduce the risk of cancer by 77%. [22 A] Stanford University breast cancer study found a strong link between reduced sun exposure and cancer incidence. Conducted on 4000 women aged 35 –79, it found that women with light skin and high sun exposure **had half the risk of developing advanced breast cancer**.[23] Other cancers that appear linked with vitamin D deficiency include colon, lung, rectum, ovary, pancreas, prostate, and multiple myeloma.

Cancer and other degenerative diseases are often called, "diseases of civilization." As we move inside from the more natural, outdoor, God-made environment we were created for, our bodies simply break down more easily.

SUN PROTECTION

Too many people live under the philosophy of:

If a little's good, a whole lot's better.

Knowing that, it's time for me to come down hard on overexposure to the sun. In extolling the benefits of the sun, I am in no way telling you to go "hog wild" on sunbathing. Whenever I go to Hawaii, I invariably see lots of people sunbathing, some of whom look like boiled lobsters. Now that's dumber than not getting any sun at all! Though people have worked out in the sun from the beginning of human history, they've also been smart enough to protect themselves by covering up. That's why, as a very fair-skinned person, I only go to beaches in Hawaii that have shade. I get plenty of sun exposure just being in the outdoors without having to purposely bake my bare body in the tropical sun.

Proper sun exposure is good, but, as we previously discussed, sunscreen is bad. So what do you do to prevent sunburn? Here's what I suggest for sun protection:

1. Limit Exposure – Get no more than 15 minutes of midday summer sun exposure per day. Then cover up or get into the shade. This is your best protection.

2. Dietary Change – Avoiding all polyunsaturated fats is essential. This would include safflower, corn and soy oils. Instead use healthy saturated fats like virgin coconut oil and butter and, to a lesser extent, monounsaturated fats such as olive oil. Your skin is only damaged by normal sun exposure when your body lacks the antioxidants needed to protect the cells. The Standard American Diet (SAD Diet) doesn't help at this point. Most junk food robs your cells of oxygen – fried foods being especially harmful. So dump the French fries and donuts!

3. Supplementation – The amino acid L-tyrosine is a precursor for the formation of the melanin pigment in the skin. Thus, an adequate level of this nutrient is key to sun protection. Copper, vitamin B-6 and vitamin C work synergistically with tyrosine, and thus may also be helpful nutrients. Jonathan Wright, M.D., recommends the following nutritional supplementation before sun exposure: [24]

1000 – 1500 mg L-tyrosine

1000 – 1500 mg Vitamin C

50 mg Vitamin B-6

4 mg Copper (2 – 3 weeks in advance of going on vacation)

30 mg Zinc Citrate or Picolinate while taking the copper.

Folic Acid, vitamin B-12 and vitamin A may also be helpful as antioxidants that aid in cell reproduction and repair.

4. Natural Sunscreens – Are there "natural sunscreens" products that will prevent sunburn? Yes. If you can't avoid overexposure to sun, such as on a beach or hiking, there are some more natural alternatives to the toxic chemical sunscreens. Health food stores carry such products. Look for natural sunscreens containing titanium dioxide, which has the effect of deflecting UV radiation off the skin. Some other products feature Green Tea for its antioxidant value.

Some of the latest findings indicate an extract made from broccoli sprouts may protect against skin cancer. Broccoli, and especially its sprouts, contains sulphoraphane, which stimulates anti-cancer activity in the cells. Researchers found 37% less redness on UV exposed areas of the skin covered with the broccoli extract. Rather than just deflecting the UV radiation, the broccoli extract goes down deep into the skin producing a resistance to cancer formation.[25] Though no product is yet available to the public using broccoli extract, look for this in the future.

CONCLUSION

The point is simple: the sun is good for you in the right amount. It's unhealthy to avoid the sun altogether. It's also unhealthy to be overexposed to the sun and get sunburn. Like most areas of life, sun exposure is about discovering the right balance. Plan to get limited exposure to natural sunlight for 15 minutes a day. In the winter months, when the sun isn't as effective, supplement with vitamin D-

3. Recognizing it as the key to all life, and let the sun enhance your life and health. You'll feel better, you'll look better, and according to the research, and you'll reduce your risk of many common diseases.

Chapter 6

Sleep That Satisfies

. . . that one may sleep satisfied . . . (Proverbs 19:23, NASB)

A Gallup Poll commissioned by the National Sleep Foundation found that one out of every two people suffers from sleeplessness at some point in their lives. As many as 40 million Americans suffer from serious sleep disorders that affect not only their sleep quality, but their overall health. During the 20th century, the average amount of time asleep has been reduced by 20 percent, and in the past 25 years, we've added the equivalent of *one month* to our average annual work and commute time. We're **working longer and sleeping less.**

COST OF SLEEP PROBLEMS

People who get enough sleep find they have greater productivity and attentiveness, making it easier to handle minor problems and irritations. Conversely, sleep problems frequently caused strained relationships at home and work. Sufferers of chronic insomnia are more likely to need healthcare services and specifically to develop psychiatric problems. Every year in America fatigue is blamed for 200,000 car accidents.

In a message to pastors the great English preacher Charles Spurgeon said:

> *. . . I am emotionally less resilient when I lose sleep. There were early days when I would work without regard to sleep and feel energized and motivated. In the last seven or eight years my threshold for despondency is much lower. For me, adequate sleep is not a matter of staying healthy. It is a*

matter of staying in the ministry. It is irrational that my future should look bleaker when I get four or five hours sleep several nights in a row. But that is irrelevant. Those are the facts. And I must live within the limits of facts. I commend sufficient sleep to you, for the sake of your proper assessment of God and His promises.

HOW MUCH SLEEP IS ENOUGH?

When it comes to the question of how much sleep one really needs, there may be as many opinions as people. While I can go along with the idea that the amount of sleep needed varies between individuals, I still think there are minimums that apply to virtually anyone. I cannot imagine that six hours of sleep over a prolonged period of time is enough for anyone, though there are some who say even four hours *may* be enough for some individuals. The same experts will also say, however, that ten hours *are not enough* for other individuals.

Babies sleep for about 17 hours per day, which reduces to nine to ten hours for older children. I think it's safe to say that most adults need at least seven to eight hours of sleep per night. Many authorities feel that elderly people need less sleep, but this may be in part related to naps being taken during the day. Other authorities, whom I'm more inclined to agree with, disagree noting that our bodies are *less able to sustain sleep* than when they were younger. Older people need the sleep — they just have trouble getting it.

YOU NEED MORE SLEEP IF . . .

Instead of debating the ideal or minimum amount of sleep *everyone* needs, I think it's more helpful to look at **symptoms that indicate that you need more sleep:**

1. Do you have trouble staying awake during boring or monotonous situations (lectures, meetings, church, routine work, driving)?

2. Do you have difficulty concentrating or remembering facts?

3. Do you have problems with making decisions?

4. Are you frequently depressed, irritable or moody?

If any of the above describes you, there's a good chance you're not getting enough sleep, *even if you're getting eight or more hour.* Conversely, you can experiment with sleeping more hours to see if you feel better.

THE SLEEP PROCESS

Sleep begins with Stage One, a light sleep, wherein your muscles relax and your brain waves are irregular and rapid. In Stage Two sleep the brain waves become larger and are characterized by bursts of electrical activity. Stages Three and Four involve deep sleep, in which large slow brain waves (sometimes called delta waves) are produced.

After an hour or so REM (rapid eye movement) sleep begins. This is the dreaming stage during which your brain waves are similar to the waking state. REM sleep typically occurs several times during the night. About 75% of the night is spent in non-REM sleep and 25% in REM sleep, with the REM periods getting longer and more frequent as the night goes on.

SLEEP DISORDERS

1. Insomnia —Insomnia is trouble falling asleep *or* staying asleep. It also affects waking hours with sleepiness or trouble concentrating. Insomnia can be *transient* (difficulty sleeping for a few nights due to excitement, stress, time zone changes, etc.), *short-term* (two to three weeks from longer periods of work or home stress), or *chronic* (ongoing insomnia).

Causes may include stress, stimulant usage, nicotine or other drug usage, psychiatric disorders, unusual hours, inactive behavior, noise or light interference, arthritic or other pain, overuse of sleeping pills, gastric reflux, unstopped brain activity, nutrient deficiencies, and more.

2. Narcolepsy —Narcolepsy refers to a chronic, frequent, irresistible need to sleep. These "sleep attacks" can happen at any time without warning and last for anywhere from seconds to a half hour. In narcolepsy the victim goes into a sudden onset of REM sleep. This, of course, is particularly dangerous if you're driving a car or operating machinery. Other symptoms that may be experienced include cataplexy (loss of muscle function), sleep paralysis (temporary inability to move the body when falling asleep or waking), and hypnagogic hallucinations (vivid, dream-like, frightening experiences when first falling asleep).

About 50,000 Americans have been diagnosed with narcolepsy, though 200,000 are believed to be affected. Conventional medicine says the cause is unknown. Personally, I feel that chronic boredom or need to escape stressful situations must play a role in this problem. I've never met a mentally active, goal-oriented, driven, happy person with narcolepsy.

3. Sleep Apnea —Over ten million Americans don't breathe properly when they sleep. This causes an oxygen deficiency, poor sleep, daytime sleepiness, and increased risk of cardiovascular problems. Loud snoring is the primary indicator of a possible sleep apnea problem — 30% of adults snore, but this is only serious for about 5% of them.

There are two types of sleep apnea: *Obstructive Sleep Apnea* is the most common and the most dangerous type. When the muscles of the soft palate relax and sag, the airway is blocked making breathing labored and noisy. Ten to 60 seconds may elapse between loud snores with deep gasps for air as the breathing starts. Most often obstructive sleep apnea is a problem of overweight men.

Central Sleep Apnea relates to the brain signal to breathe being delayed. This is usually a less serious problem that manifests itself with increasing age, with one in four people over age 60 experiencing it.

4. Restless Leg Syndrome (RLS) —With this disorder creeping, crawling, tingling or painful sensations occur primarily in the calf, but may affect the whole leg. Symptoms are most common when lying or sitting for a long time and are usually worse at night. Sufferers feel an urge to move the legs and experience some relief from moving, walking or massaging the legs.

Ever heard of "growing pains?" That's a form of RLS in children, as is some hyperactivity. If your child has "growing pains," something's wrong, because **growth doesn't hurt!** Mineral deficiencies, especially magnesium, are the most likely causes.

5. Periodic Leg Movement Disorder (PLMD) —Unlike RLS movements which are voluntary, PLMD movements are involuntary, most often occurring during sleep. It's estimated that 35% or more of those over 65 experience this disorder. This jerking of the legs during sleep again may be connected with mineral deficiencies, especially magnesium.

6. Delayed Sleep Phase Syndrome (DSPS) —This is believed to be a "biological clock" disorder related to the body's circadian rhythm. Someone with DSPS has difficulty falling asleep and waking up because their body clock doesn't fit with their desired sleep and wake times. It's like jet lag or time zone travel that is longer lasting.

About half the DSPS sufferers also experience depression. This may stem in part from being different from everyone else. Going to bed earlier and trying to get up earlier usually just fuels their frustration. Sleeping pills don't help and may make the problem worse.

GENERAL SUGGESTIONS

1. Avoid caffeine

2. Avoid alcohol and nicotine.

3. Exercise regularly – not too close to bedtime.

4. Get up at the same time daily regardless of when you went to bed the night before.

5. Fix bedroom problems with light, noise, heat or cold.

6. Don't eat a heavy meal within three hours of bedtime.

7. Avoid using sleeping pills.

8. Establish a "winding down" routine for bedtime.

9. Don't "try hard" to go to sleep or get frustrated about not going to sleep. Do something till you get tired.

NATURAL MEDICINE APPROACHES

While there are specific natural medicine approaches to help sleep problems, the most important approach, as always, is the **fix the basics.** Correcting nutrient deficiencies, allergic sensitivities and toxicities in the general sense will help or eliminate many sleep problems. Other possibilities include:

1. High Magnesium Multi-Mineral —Though extra chelated magnesium by itself is sometimes appropriate, I generally prefer a multi-mineral with extra magnesium. Magnesium is a relaxer, and helps with many sleep problems.

2. Melatonin —The pineal gland hormone melatonin has gotten a lot of publicity, and rightly so — but it isn't for everyone. Melatonin governs the body's time clock in relationship to light and darkness. Therefore it can especially be helpful for sleep problems like Delayed Sleep Phase Syndrome, jet lag and the like. Some people react to melatonin with feelings of grogginess upon awakening, or vivid, disturbing dreams. Individual testing, as done at my clinic, will indicate if you need melatonin.

We are consistently finding that melatonin-herbal combinations test better and work better than straight melatonin, at least for most individuals. We also occasionally use melatonin, serotonin, and dopamine homeopathic formulas.

3. Herbs —Valerian, or combinations with valerian, scullcap, passion flower, hops and other relaxing herbs may help on sleep.

4. Phosphatidyl Serine —This product can be helpful for people too hyper to go to sleep. It is oriented toward reducing high levels of adrenal hormones in the evening that otherwise interfere with normal sleep.

5. L-Tryptophan or 5-Hydroxy-Tryptophan —This is a precursor to serotonin and can help with sleep. Foods high in tryptophan that might be tried at bedtime include turkey, bananas, figs, dates, yogurt, tuna, whole grain crackers, and nut butter.

Have a good night!

Chapter 7

Healthy Attitudes

. . . have this attitude . . . (Philippians 3:15, NASB)

The right attitude is the key to almost everything in life —and health is no exception. It might be better to say "attitudes" rather than just "attitude," since there are numerous mental orientations that comprise good health. In Proverbs we're told,

As a man thinketh in his heart, so is he. (Prov. 23:7, KJV)

And it's true! What we think really does determine who and what we are. But how does this apply to health? What attitudes do we really need to adopt to enhance our health? Though there are undoubtedly more than I have thought of, here's a beginning:

#1 COMMITMENT

Commitment is at the top of my list, simply because I observe this attitude consistently in my clients making the most dramatic progress. The people who get the best results in solving their health problems generally approach those problems with the greatest resolve. They are committed to dietary changes, the nutritional supplements, exercise, adequate sleep, or about whatever else I suggest. They have taken control, *and* they have taken responsibility.

Remember the story of Jesus and the paralytic at the Pool of Bethesda? It says:

> *And a certain man was there, who had been thirty-eight years* **in his sickness.** *When Jesus saw him lying there, and knew that he had already been a long time in that condition, He said to him,* **"Do you wish to get well?"** (John 5:5-6, NASB)

I think there's more in this passage than meets the eye — don't be fooled by the simplicity of the story. Note that the passage says (most literally translated in the *New American Standard Bible) not* that the man had been sick for thirty-eight years, *but* that he had been *in his sickness* for thirty-eight years. It wasn't just that his sickness was in him, but that he was in his sickness – a much greater problem! Furthermore, I think Jesus words that follow corroborate this interpretation.

It says Jesus knew he had been there that way for a long time (some Bible scholars believe the length of the man's illness is symbolic of Israel's wilderness wanderings), yet asks him the most unusual question of whether or not he wanted to get well. I can't think of another encounter quite like that in Scripture. We can only conclude that Jesus felt the man was committed not to health, but to remaining sick.

This is further proven by the paralytic's response — an excuse. Why, he couldn't be healed because he had no one to put him in the water at the moment the angel stirred the water. Come off of it! In thirty-eight years he couldn't find someone to put him in the water? Lame! Lame! Lame! He was just not committed, preferring to wallow in self-pity instead. But Jesus had other plans, as hopefully He does for you too.

Someone committed to health (which means being committed to change) will follow any diet, stop eating any problem food or beverage, take any supplement, follow any exercise program . . . they will do whatever it takes. Jesus taught us: "Knock and it shall be opened;" "Seek and you shall find."

#2 SELF-DISCIPLINE

In Galatians 5:22-23 we read that self-control or self-discipline is one of the nine fruit of the Spirit. In other words, this is an attribute that *should* be the result of being filled and controlled by the Holy Spirit. In fact, it's listed as the last fruit, the last position always having a special importance. The Spirit's control in your life begins with love and ends with self-control . . . but few Christians really experience that.

I've found it humorous over my 40 plus year association with Christian ministry to occasionally have certain Christians look down their nose at me because I didn't share their particular ecstatic spiritual gift. But they often lacked the *real* fruit of the Spirit, self-discipline, as did their churches full of gluttonous people!

How do you develop this attitude of self-discipline in our indulgent, "if it feels good, do it" world? The first suggestion I would have is fasting. Regular, plain water, fasting has an awesome ability to break the connection we enjoy with fulfilling our desires and impulses versus fulfilling God's desires. It truly builds self-discipline.

But fasting isn't just a principle that works relative to food. You can fast from TV, or other distractions as well in order to sharpen your sensitivities and reinforce your own discipline.

#3 POSITIVE ATTITUDE

Though worldly success teachers make much of positive mental attitude, Christians would do well to learn their lessons. I can think of no better illustration of positive mental attitude than a half glass of water. One person looks at it and says it's half full, while the other person looks at it and says its half empty. Guess which one has the positive mental attitude?

Now this isn't just a matter of opinion. Think about it — the only **reality** inside the glass is the water. The empty space in the other half is just that —**nothing!** You aren't just negative if you're focused on the nothing half, but rather are deceived.

Every situation may be looked at by the Christian as having positive value . . . because of the ***promises of God.*** He said, "In everything give thanks" (I Thessalonians 5:18) — it wasn't just Pollyanna's idea. And you can do that as a Christian because God is in control, He is sovereign and therefore Romans 8:28 may be claimed:

> *He causes all things to work together for good to those who love Him, to those called according to His purpose.*

Sometimes I think we miss the depth of what Romans 8:28 is really saying. R. C. Sproul notes that this teaches that **nothing *ultimately* bad can happen to a believer** who (1) loves God, and (2) is called according to his purpose. Though many things happen that seem *proximately* bad, that is, bad in the near-term, everything in your life as a committed believer will *ultimately* be good. What an amazing promise to lay hold of!

#4 GOAL ORIENTATION

If you're committed, disciplined and positive, you tend to want and have goals. Now I don't just mean "health" goals. A goal-orientation in your life overall is health producing. A lack of goal-orientation is self-destructive. Let me illustrate:

Let's say an ICBM missile is fired at an enemy target. That missile has a guidance mechanism in it that knows where it's going — that is to say, it has a pre-programmed **goal.** If that guidance system fails, if the missile is off-course, it no longer has its goal. That's very dangerous, so we have a **self-destruct button** that the controllers will push. People are about the same — only when we have no goals, we push our own self-destruct button. It's seldom outright suicide, but the result is the same — premature death.

#5 PATIENCE

Patience, like self-discipline, is the fruit of the Holy Spirit in our lives. If we really know who God is, if we know His omnipotence, omniscience, goodness, mercy and sovereignty, what else can we do but be patient with the working out of His plan? Life is characterized largely by a lot of trials, a lot of suffering. In James 1:2-4 we're told:

> *Consider it all joy, my brethren, when you encounter various trials, knowing that the testing of your faith produces endurance (i.e. patience); and let endurance have its perfect result, that you may be perfect (i.e. mature, whole), lacking in nothing.*

#6 PEACE

What do you know — it's another fruit of the Spirit. Peace tends to flow from these other attitudes as we understand God's control. If you're in control of your life, you won't have much peace. But if God's in control, peace is the natural, or should I say *supernatural,* result.

Many people with chronic health problems have no peace. The person at peace knows that the worst thing that can happen to them health-wise is dying — and in reality, death is the best thing that can happen to a Christian — it's our graduation ceremony!

#7 FEARLESSNESS

The absence of fear likewise results from knowing the sovereign God and His control in your life. Few things rob you of life and health more than fear. Are you obsessed with constant worry about everyone and everything? Then you're not walking in God's Spirit. To the extent that you worry, to that same extent you are not trusting God. Paul wrote:

> *Be anxious for nothing, but in everything, by prayer and supplication with thanksgiving, let your requests be made known to God.* (Philippians 4:6)

The only thing you need to fear is God . . . and then you don't need to fear anyone or anything else.

#8 FORGIVENESS

Few things are more healing than simple forgiveness. I would suggest that anyone with a health problem make a list of the people you've held something against, that you harbor bitterness against, and forgive them. Forgive them because God commands, but also forgive them because it's part of your spiritual *and* physical healing as well. Professor Lewis Smedes said:

> *To forgive is to set a prisoner free and discover that the prisoner was you.*

#9 TEACHABILITY

Do you ever wonder why Jesus picked the disciples? They were a pretty motley crew — a wide range of education, occupations, temperaments, and the like. What was the common denominator? The only one I can find is teachability. The only **ability** that really counts in life is **teachability**— being willing to learn, from God, from yourself and from others.

To be healthy you're going to have to learn a lot that's contrary to your present thinking, to the way you were brought up, to the way your friends and family think. Health is about change, and you won't change unless you're teachable.

#10 HUMILITY

I saved this one for last. Humility ties all these healthy attitudes together. When we approach life understanding our pitiful condition without God's grace, humility is the only reasonable response . . . and humility heals from the inside out. If you truly understand your condition before receiving God's grace that drew you to faith, you'll have nothing to be proud about. We were all part of a race of traitors and rebels against God's throne, spiritually dead with no hope of regaining that spiritual life and relationship with God. Paul describes our "Before Christ" condition this way:

> *And you were dead in the trespasses and sin in which you once walked, following the course of this world, following the prince of the power of the air, the spirit that is now at work in the sons of disobedience—among whom we all once lived in the passions of our flesh, carrying out the desires of the body and the mind, and were by nature children of wrath, like the rest of mankind.* (Ephesians 2:1-3)

But then he adds our "After Christ" position in the next verse:

> *But God, being rich in mercy, because of the great love with which he loved us, even when we were dead in our trespasses, made us alive together with Christ—by grace you have been saved . . .* (Ephesians 2:4-5)

If we really understand who we "were" before and who "are" now in Christ, humility is the only reasonable response. Pride destroys; humility heals.

Chapter 8

Capturing the Present Moment

. . . forgetting what lies behind, I press on . . . (Philippians 3:14)

It was a cold, rainy December night in 1980. I was writing a newsletter article simply sharing the highlights of what God had taught me that past year. Many problems and frustrations I had endured came to mind, most of which I was still enduring. A lot of that frustration revolved around my cramped working space. You see, my "office" was an old eight foot travel trailer parked next to our 12 by 60 foot mobile home on a small acreage in the foothills of the Southern Oregon Cascade Range. My desk was an unstable, pull-down table. The heat was a slightly inadequate portable electric heater connected to the mobile home by a 50 foot extension cord.

I wanted in the worst way to build a house on our property, or at least an office-garage combination, yet that was financially impossible. There were other financial pressures too, like a car needing $1000 in major repairs. A major ministry employment opportunity had fallen through a few months before. About all I had was my health. You get the picture – it was a rough time.

But as those thoughts burdened my mind, the Spirit of God touched me in a very special way. The frustrations of my heart melted as I saw a principle, recently renewed in my heart that made my circumstances irrelevant. This concept produces a peace and joy that powerfully heals, resolving most emotional stress . . . if we let it. I call this concept **capturing the present moment.**

IN WHAT MOMENT DO YOU LIVE?

You can only live in three possible "moments" – the *past* moment, the *future* moment, or the *present* moment. If you're like most people, you'll immediately say:

Sure I live in the present moment. Where else could I live?

Despite protestations to the contrary, I find very few people who consistently live in the present moment. Most are imprisoned in either their past failures or their anticipated future glories. Either one represents considerable bondage. Jesus came to proclaim liberty to the captives (Luke 4:18), so let's see if this concept can release you from any mental prisons that are creating holes in your wholeness. To better understand the "present moment," we need to first examine the "past moment" and "future moment."

THE PAST MOMENT – "If only I had . . ."

The word most characterizing the past moment is *guilt*. How often, how incredibly often do you look back with "if only" statements? Do you regurgitate the past saying, "If only I had done this," or "If only I had not done that?" Do you entertain that persistent illusion that your life would be so much better – if only? That thinking, frankly, is delusional. How do you know anything would have been any different in the long run? What other even more undesirable circumstances might have occurred to have made the situation even worse? You don't know. You cannot know.

The first time I remember struggling with the past moment was near the end of my second year of college campus Christian ministry when I forced my superiors to change my ministry assignment. In my lust for conquering new horizons, I was restless to move on to some different challenge than Bozeman, Montana. My ministry directors ultimately sent me to start a new work on a small campus in Missouri, where alone my wife and I spent one of the most miserable years of our lives. Like fruit picked from a tree prematurely, my spiritual maturity just wasn't happening. The end of that year saw us moving to yet another ministry assignment with a new problem – I had cancer.

At the time it looked like one domino after another had fallen since that one bad decision. The only factor left out of my thought process was God. My lament could only continue until I saw God in the picture. Was he there? Yes. Was he sovereignly working through the decision I made, no matter how foolish they seem to me now? Yes. Did he use all of my decisions as part of his design to channel my life in the direction he had planned? Yes. Have all the mistakes in my life been used to bring me to exactly where he wants me in this present moment? Yes. And thus a past moment fades away as a present moment is captured.

Retrospectively, I now have an entirely different view of that situation. I wouldn't be writing this book (and you wouldn't be reading it) if I hadn't made that "error." That chain of events ultimately moved me from a ministry I wasn't suited for anyway to now 30 years as an alternative health care practitioner. Back then, I overvalued my mistakes because I erroneously thought I was in the driver's seat of my life. I now realize that not only was I not in the driver's seat, but I didn't even know the destination. And neither do you.

I could fill a whole book with other examples from my life – of homes purchased that shouldn't have been, of moves made that shouldn't have been, of employment opportunities that should or shouldn't have been taken, of money that shouldn't have been borrowed, of businesses that shouldn't have been started, of cars that shouldn't have been bought and on and on. But all of these experiences evaporate into insignificance once the God who "works all things together for good" comes on the scene in my mind. Once I again see and believe that he really does provide for *all* my needs, I am free from the torture of the past – I have captured the present moment.

"MEDITATING" ON FAILURE

How many past failures do you "meditate" on? Yes, meditating is really what it is – literally, chewing the cud. If you haven't been around cud-chewing animals (ruminants) like cows, sheep or goats, let me educate you. Ruminants have four stomachs – the reticulum, rumen, omasum and abomasum. After a lot of chewing the food initially goes into the reticulum. It's then regurgitated up for further chewing and goes to the rumen for more digestion. The process continues until the animals fully digest its food.

We swallow that failure when it originally occurred, but then we keep bringing it up to chew on it some more in what becomes a hopeless attempt to digest it. By contrast the Bible tells us to meditate on God's Word and his promises of life, peace, perspective, and prosperity. Meditate on anything else, including past failures, and you are doomed to emotional indigestion (and probably physical indigestion too). Meditating on failure is guaranteed to drain the life right out of you.

REMEMBER WHEN

Another variation of living in the past moment is "living in the good ol' days." I got a more than healthy dose of this growing up. Though my father died in 1998, I think his calendar stopped in about 1948. He constantly hearkened back to some earlier time when things seemed so much better. He must have been a good teacher, since I've done a lot of "remembering when" in my own life. How often, amidst huge trials, I've recalled how simple my life was in college or the two summers during college when I worked at Crater Lake National Park in that idyllic setting.

Were the "good ol' days" really that good? Probably not. We easily delude ourselves with selective memory, romanticizing the glories of the past and conveniently forgetting the adversities. The truth is that those past moments are not real, they no longer exist, and their time has passed. They could only be enjoyed within their own "present moment." You can no more hold past time than you can hold water in your hand. What I'm saying is that **there really are no past moments**, other than in your own imagination. They are forever gone – for which we should thank God. The poet, Carl Sandburg, in contemplating the ruins of an ancient civilization lamented:

The past is gone forever; let the dead be dead.

I prefer the Apostle Paul's instruction, though:

> *But one thing I do: forgetting what lies behind and straining forward to what lies ahead, I press on toward the goal for the prize of the upward call of God in Christ Jesus.* (Philippians 3:13b-14)

Think of how incredible his statement is! Imagine what *he* had to forget in the past, having been the number one persecutor of the church, overseeing the murder of the church's first martyr, Stephen. Paul could have been paralyzed with guilt over his past failures and mistakes, but he chose otherwise.

ESCAPING THE PAST MOMENT

The theory's great, but how can we really escape the past and leave it behind? We can the same way Paul did: By seeing past failures hung on the cross of Christ. Your past, as well as your present and future, is what Jesus suffered and died for. Since he suffered for it so you wouldn't have to, why do you persist in trying to suffer for it yourself? Why should you or I carry around what he has already removed and dealt with? Paul wrote:

> *For you have died and your life is hidden with Christ in God.* (Colossians 3:3)

> *There is therefore now no condemnation for those who are in Christ Jesus.* (Romans 8:1)

> *We were buried therefore with him by baptism into death, in order that, just as Christ was raised from the dead by the glory of the Father, we too might walk in newness of life.* (Romans 6:4)

As we comprehend the full significance of the cross, we can escape the past moment.

THE FUTURE MOMENT – "If only I could . . . "

Most people see the problems associated with living in the *past* moment, but will justify living in the equally unproductive *future* moment. The future moment is simply a switch from preoccupation with past "if onlys" to future "if onlys." Either way, **you miss the present moment**.

Like most people I have a lot more of a problem here than with the past. It's so easy to say, "If only I had . . .

More clients

More product sales

More books published

Better investments

. . . and so on. We get the idea that when we have that future whatever, we will have it together – everything will finally be all right. But you can sooner form a ball out of sand or hold the wind in your hands than benefit from living in a future dream.

Like the past, the future is an unreal world that exists only in our minds. For once the future comes it is no longer future, but present. The mystique and fantasy fade, as it arrives in the reality of the present moment. How often we suffer disappointment as the future arrived less glorious than anticipated. Even when we exactly achieve our future goals, we get a whole new set of circumstances to contend with. The deck gets shuffled causing further frustration in spite of our achievement.

How many dream houses, dream cars, dream jobs, or dream business opportunities carry with them the burden of increased cares, responsibilities, costs, and time? More or less, all of them do. Then you experience the letdown – that hollow feeling once you get what you at least *thought* would make you happy. The inner discontent still simmers *in spite of* reaching that future goal. You graduate from college, you get a certain job or promotion, you buy a certain car, you purchase that home or second home . . . but along with them come a whole new set of trials.

I am of course describing the basic error of materialism, as was summarized with the "yuppie" bumper sticker:

> *He who has the most toys at the end of the game wins.*

Living in future materialistic dreams is doomed to failure, as Jesus taught:

> *Take care, and be on your guard against all covetousness, for one's life does not consist in the abundance of his possessions.* (Luke 12:15)

Solomon likewise echoed this sentiment:

> *He who loves money will not be satisfied with money, nor he who loves wealth with his income; this also is vanity. When goods increase, they increase who eat them, and what advantage has their owner but to see them with his eyes?* (Ecclesiastes 5:10-11)

There's really no satisfaction in the future moment, though that's where most of us spend our lives, missing the beauty of the present moment's reality and perfect provision. Solomon, perhaps as no one else in the Bible, saw the futility of desire for future accumulation, yet unfortunately he apparently never discovered the fulfillment he needed he already had:

> *And whatever my eyes desired I did not keep from them. I kept my heart from no pleasure, for my heart found pleasure in all my toil, and this was my reward for all my toil. Then I considered all that my hands had done and the toil I had expended in doing it, and behold, all was vanity and a striving after wind, and there was nothing to be gained under the sun.* (Ecclesiastes 2:10-11)

In the New Testament James brings us a similar indictment on getting too wrapped up in our future plans:

> *Come now, you who say, "Today or tomorrow we will go into such and such a town and spend a year there and trade and make a profit" – yet you do not know what tomorrow will bring. What is your life? For you are a mist that appears*

for a little time and then vanishes. Instead you ought to say, "If the Lord wills, we will live and do this or that." As it is, you boast in your arrogance. All such boasting is evil. (James 4:13-16)

Future moment living is a great enemy of contentment and the corresponding health it brings to body, mind and spirit. There's no more happiness in the future moment than there is in the past moment. Our only fulfillment can be experienced in the present moment. But we must enter in.

VALUING THE PRESENT MOMENT

Charles Spurgeon said:

> *There is no other time in which you will live. The past is gone, the future has not arrived, and you have only the present.*[1]

We find true life only in the present moment. But how do we really embrace that truth? How do we get this from head theory to heart experience? The key is **contentment** – a subject the Bible says a lot about:

> *The Lord is my chosen portion and my cup; you hold my lot. The lines have fallen for me in pleasant places; indeed, I have a beautiful inheritance.* (Psalm 16:5-6)

What a description of the contentment experienced in the present moment! When we see God as our only truly valuable asset and as our complete provision and sustenance, we see the beauty of what we have right now. In another Psalm David said:

> *Because the Lord is my Shepherd, I have everything that I need.* (Psalm 23:1 Living Bible)

The problem we often have with our present moment is we dislike the particular circumstances God has ordained. Such was the problem of the Corinthian church regarding singles wanting to be married and married people wanting to be single. Paul exhorted them to contentment with the present moment:

> *Only let each person lead the life that the Lord has assigned to him, and to which God has called him . . . Each one should remain in the condition in which he was called.* (I Corinthians 7:17a, 20)

You will never find peace in wanting to be in different circumstances. **Peace *only* flows out of contentment with *present* circumstances.** Only when you're content with the now, can God change it to a new situation to build the character of contentment in you.

EXAMPLE OF PAUL

The Apostle Paul demonstrates such a superior example of delighting in the present moment. In spite of the adversity he encountered, look at his philosophy of contentment penned from a prison cell:

> *Not that I am speaking of being in need, for I have learned in whatever situation I am to be content. I know how to be brought low, and I know how to abound. In any and every circumstance, I have learned the secret of facing plenty and hunger, abundance and need. I can do all things through him who strengthens me.* (Philippians 4:11-13)

What is he saying to us? Simply that he had learned the secret of living in the present moment, regardless of his circumstances. Since God was in his present moment, that's where Paul chose to live and experience contentment.

Paul also saw contentment as the validation of true godliness:

> *Now there is great gain in godliness with contentment, for we brought nothing into the world, and we cannot take anything out of the world. But if we have food and clothing, with these we will be content.* (I Timothy 6:6-8)

Note that he only gives two basic material essentials for contentment – food and clothing. Nothing about houses, cars, employment, education or a dozen other things we usually view as essentials for contentment. What if you just made a decision that food and clothing were all you absolutely had to have and everything else was just icing on the cake? Do you think that would make it easier to capture the present moment? It works for me.

The author of Hebrews pens a similar exhortation:

> *Keep your life free from love of money, and be content with what you have, for he has said, "I will never leave you nor forsake you." So we can confidently say, "The Lord is my helper; I will not fear; what can man do to me?"* (Hebrews 13:5-6)

Ultimately we must see that God alone is the sole ingredient necessary for our happiness and fulfillment. And guess what? He operates, not in the vapors of the past or future, but only in the "now" of our lives – in the present moment.

6 STEPS TO THE PRESENT MOMENT

Let's get practical. How do you really go about capturing the present moment? That answer is a little different for everyone, but there are some general biblical principles that apply to all of us. Here are six steps to point you in the right direction:

1. Fully Accept Your Past, Present and Future

You'll never step into the present until you make peace with your past. You can't deny your past, nor can you change it. Acceptance is therefore the only alternative. God told Jeremiah:

> *Before I formed you in the womb I knew you, and before you were born I consecrated you; I appointed you a prophet to the nations.* (Jeremiah 1:5)

Everything in Jeremiah's life, and even before his conception, was known and foreordained by God. Does Jeremiah respond to this declaration with praise to God and contentment? No. Instead, he lives in the past moment, bemoaning his faults:

Alas, Lord God! Behold, I do not know how to speak, because I am a youth. (Jeremiah 1:6)

Dare you apply this scripture to yourself? God's hand has likewise been on you from before your beginning. Just as Jeremiah's inabilities were part of God's curriculum, so your past is preparatory as well. Look back at the past (especially all your mistakes) like a military boot camp. Though it was hell to go through, and you don't have to repeat it – it was fundamental preparation to the battles ahead. Remember that, above all, tragedies and triumphs of the past are a profound testimony of the grace of God working in your life. When you see them as such, the peace treaty with your past will be signed and ratified.

How about fully accepting the present? Here's a key: **See your present as being okay for your current level of maturity.** Would you expect a two week old child to walk? Of course not. That would be beyond his or her level of maturity. Are you perhaps too spiritually young and immature to expect perfection from? Your present condition is where God has brought you to thus far. It isn't the final destination, for he has promised to continue to mature you into his image (Philippians 1:6). Therefore, don't bemoan your present circumstances, but rather see them as perfect for where God has you and what he is doing in your life *today*. See today's adversity as a step down the path toward maturity. See yourself as right on schedule because the omnipotent and sovereign God is in charge of the process.

In the same spirit we need to accept our unknown future. Have you ever experienced the stress of driving your car on a dark and rainy night to a hard to find address? Compare that with sitting in the back seat with someone else driving who knows exactly where the destination is, having been there before. You may think that you are behind the steering wheel, but in reality you're just a passenger with Jesus doing the driving. Relax and let him take you to his desired destination. See your future as something you really can't control, but that you can trust God to complete. He really has the best plan.

2. Welcome Trials

Living in the present moment is only possible if you can accept any possible circumstance. Can you welcome trials? Can you actually *love* trials, knowing their higher value? If you hate difficult circumstances that land in your life, you will either shift into the past moment or into the future moment. *Hating trials prohibits living in the present moment.*

Trials are not easy. You have to have a reason, a very good reason, for *loving* trials. The biblical motivation for welcoming trials is in simply knowing the benefits they produce. Let's look at a few passages:

> *When all kinds of trials and temptations crowd into your lives, my brothers, don't resent them as intruders, but welcome them as friends! Realize that they come to test your faith and to produce in you the quality of endurance. But let the process go on until that endurance is fully developed, and you will find you have become men of mature character with the right sort of independence.* (James 1:2-4, Philips)

> *We can rejoice, too, when we run into problems and trials for we know that they are good for us – they help us learn to be patient. And patience develops strength of character in us and helps us trust God more each time we use it until finally our hope and faith are strong and steady. Then, when that happens, we are able to hold our heads high no matter what happens and know that all is well, for we know how dearly God loves us, and we feel this warm love everywhere within us because God has given us the Holy Spirit to fill our hearts with his love.* (Romans 5:3-5, Living Bible)

> *So be truly glad! There is wonderful joy ahead, even though the going is rough for a while down here. These trials are only to test your faith, to see whether or not it is strong, and pure. It is being tested as fire tests gold and purifies it – and your faith is far more precious to God than mere gold; so if your faith remains strong after being tried in the test tube of fiery trials, it will bring you much praise and glory, and honor on the day of his return.* (I Peter 1:6-7, Living Bible)

Dear friends, don't be bewildered or surprised when you go through the fiery trials ahead, for this is no strange, unusual thing that is going to happen to you. Instead, be really glad – because these trials will make you partners with Christ in his suffering, and afterwards you will have the wonderful joy of sharing his glory in that coming day when it will be displayed. (I Peter 4:12-13, Living Bible)

What could I say about the incredible benefits of trials that God's word has not already said? Practically his whole design for the Christian life revolves around trials. They build character, they mature, they purify, they take away the desire for sin, and they identify us with Christ, preparing us for our future inheritance. There is no greater fulfillment available in life than knowing and doing God's will – and trials lead us toward that end. A. W. Tozer said,

Before God can use a man greatly, he must first wound him deeply.

3. Focus on Basic Needs

A third step in capturing the present moment is to focus your attention on basic needs. In the Lord's Prayer we were taught to pray, "Give us this day our daily bread." That's a basic need. Earlier I referred to I Timothy 6:8 where Paul instructs us to be content with food and clothing. Have you ever suffered despondency because you lacked those two commodities? Probably not. It's all the other junk that we don't have that bothers us. Why not make a decision before God like this:

Lord, I commit myself to be content and thankful as long as you provide my basic food, clothing and shelter. I commit myself to the simple enjoyment of those basic needs.

There is such a store of happiness at that simple level, beyond which an often insatiable desire for more and more crowds out contentment.

4. Worry Short-Term

I have to confess that I worry long-term; I'll bet you do too. Instead of limiting our concerns to the immediate future, we worry months, years and even decades out. Ask yourself:

> *What concerns am I turning over in my mind right now that pertain to tomorrow, next week, next month, next year, or many years from now?*

Jesus said:

> *Therefore do not be anxious about tomorrow, for tomorrow will be anxious for itself. Sufficient for the day is its own trouble.* (Matthew 6:34)

Though few fiction characters disgust us as much as Scarlett O'Hara, she inadvertently expresses this healthy attitude in the closing lines of *Gone with the Wind*:

> *I'll think of it all tomorrow, at Tara. I can stand it then . . . After all, tomorrow is another day.*

That's how Scarlett kept her sanity, and that's how you can keep yours too. You really don't have to solve all of your problems today. You plan ahead, acknowledging, "If God wills," but you don't worry ahead. *Plan long-term, but worry short-term.*

5. Yield to God's Perfect Timing

Solomon wrote in Ecclesiastes that there was a time for everything – living, dying, killing, healing, weeping, laughing, mourning and dancing. When we know that all of our times are in the hands of a sovereign God, there is a time for everything. Peter wrote:

> *Humble yourselves, therefore, under the mighty hand of God so that at the proper time he may exalt you, casting all your anxieties on him, because he cares for you. (I Peter 5:6-7)*

Trials have a limit -- they are controlled by God's perfect timing. Your affliction will not last a second longer than necessary for it to accomplish the Father's purposes in your life. Yield to the knowledge of that perfect timing instead of fighting it.

6. Build Enjoyment into Each Day

If you capture the present moment, you can't help but enjoy life. Do you do anything each day just for your own enjoyment? "Oh, that's too self-centered," you say? "Baloney," I say! There's nothing more self-centered than slowly committing suicide by being so preoccupied with your problems that you can't pull back for a few minutes and enjoy the blessing and wonders of God and the world He's made. The sickest people I see in my practice are people who do nothing for fun. Instead of being the luscious fruit God intended their lives to be, they are like a shriveled prune.

In God's grace, seeking him and his righteousness with all your heart, you really are free to enjoy yourself. There is no biblical prohibition on it. In fact, joy is the fruit of the Holy Spirit – a fruit only borne in the present moment.

Chapter 9

Resolving Emotional Stress

. . . do not be anxious about your life . . . (Matthew 6:25a)

It can be argued that the most powerful ingredient for optimum health is the **absence of emotional stress.** Solomon said in Proverbs 17:22:

> *A joyful heart is good medicine, but a broken spirit dries up the bones.*

It is not uncommon to find people who are eating a nutritious diet, taking good nutritional supplements, exercising . . . and yet who are experiencing poor health. Unresolved emotional stress is often the "missing ingredient."

That was my experience. At the ripe old age of 24, I was told I had a serious cancer condition requiring immediate surgery, which was followed by several weeks of agonizing cobalt radiation "therapy." Though I became involved in writing and speaking and ultimately clinical practice as a result of having cancer, I was already quite "into" nutrition *before* developing the disease. For nearly two years prior we had strictly avoided refined sugar, refined flour, foods with additives, and taken all kinds of vitamins, including the ones that are supposed to prevent cancer. But the factor of emotional stress was a whole other issue that I had *not* dealt with. The following emotionally traumatic events had taken place in the months prior to the discovery of my tumor:

> 1. My wife and I were working in a college campus ministry on a new campus by ourselves. I was frustrated with not having the support personnel I had requested, with an awkward and distant relationship with my superior, and I just wasn't able to develop the commitment I desired from the students I was working with.

2. At the end of the school year I asked for another assignment, but was kept up in the air for several months on the verdict.

3. After finally finding out our destination mid-summer, we then had to move cross country.

4. After storing our furniture and belongings in the new city in southern California (we didn't have a house yet), we then traveled to Oregon to work on raising our financial support (it was a faith ministry).

5. The financial support raising was not going well in Oregon, and it was during this time that I first felt the lump, but then it seemed to go away.

6. The next month we returned to Southern California to move into our rented house and start a job that hadn't even been defined yet. Our only close friends were out of town, and we felt very disoriented and alone. It was then that the lump reappeared and I went to the doctor.

There was a whole progression of events that led up to my tumor, really one emotional trauma after another. The emotional stress that I wasn't handling well was literally eating away at me in the form of cancer.

In this chapter I want to look at the role of emotional stress in health, the mechanics of how stress is deposited, how stress defeats nutrition and detoxification, some of the common health problems produced by emotional stress, and how God liberates us from stress.

ROLE OF EMOTIONAL STRESS

The statistics on emotional stress and health are pretty incredible. The Ochsner Clinic in New Orleans found that in 500 consecutive cases of gastro-intestinal illness, *74% were caused by emotional stress.* The Yale University Out Patient Medical Dept. found *76%* of its cases were related to *emotionally induced illness.* In his best-selling book, *How to Live 365 Days a Year*, John Schindler, M.D. said that, "Three out of every four hospital beds are occupied by people with emotionally induced illness," leading him to conclude that, "Emotional stress is today our Number One cause of ill-health."

Let me hasten to add that when I talk about an illness being "emotionally induced," I'm *not* saying the symptoms are imaginary. The symptoms are very real and very physical. What we're talking about is the way emotional stress affects the physical body to produce those physical symptoms.

MAN'S FALL INTO EMOTIONAL STRESS

We find an interesting progression in the Bible that explains how emotional stress becomes such a major health problem. It's a matter of looking at what happened to the total person of Adam – body, mind and spirit – as a result of the Fall. Adam fell first in his spirit, where he lost his relationship with God through sin. *As a result* his mind was affected in that we see the entrance of destructive emotions into the human race. One of his sons in envy and anger killed his brother. Those emotions didn't exist before Adam fell in his spirit. The physical body was ultimately affected in that it ultimately experienced death.

So the progression still goes on today – from the spiritual to the emotional to the physical. Physical health problems can ultimately be traced back to emotional and spiritual origins. The Bible integrates all three together when it comes to healing:

> *My son give attention to my words; incline your ear to my sayings. Do not let them depart from your sight; keep them in the midst of your heart. For they are life to those who find them, and health to all their whole body.* (Proverbs 4:20-22, NASB)

Total healing requires dealing with the total person.

EMOTIONAL STRESS DEPOSITION

Emotional stress gets "deposited" in our bodies. To understand this, let's go back to the Creation. God created us to handle **physical** stresses. For example, if you eat some tainted food, you will either vomit it out one end or send it out the other end via diarrhea. We have **physical exhaust pipes.**

But emotional stress is a different matter because our bodies were *not* created to handle that —**we have no emotional exhaust pipes.** That's because there was no emotional stress in the original creation . . . the negative emotions of anger, guilt, fear, anxiety and the like were the result of man's Fall into sin, which came later. In the Garden there was no need for emotional exhaust pipes.

So what happens if your body doesn't have a mechanism for getting rid of emotional stress? **It gets deposited instead**— in some organ, gland, or muscle. Of all the areas in the body, it is the colon, the large intestine, that seems to be the favorite dumping ground. Dr. Schindler said:

> *The colon, more than any other organ, is a manifestor of the emotions. So much so that a wise doctor in Philadelphia remarked some years ago that "the colon is the mirror of the mind, and when the mind gets tight, the colon gets tight."*

Unfortunately the same part of your body will tend to be affected by the same stress, time and again. Dr. C. S. Lovett, in his book, *Jesus Wants You Well*, wrote:

> *Once the brain (unconscious portion) selects an organ of the body as the whipping boy for a particular emotional problem, the choice is entered into the body's computer system . . . After that, every time those same feelings occur and have to be disposed of, the stress will be directed against the SAME ORGAN . . . Consequently every organ, muscle and gland in the body could end up as a punching bag for a specific emotional problem.*

PITUITARY AND ADRENAL HORMONES

Two pituitary hormones get involved in this process —**STH** (somatotrophic hormone) and **ACTH** (adrenocorticotrophic hormone). STH mobilizes the body's defenses against infection, but in the process also produces the symptoms of what we call "sickness" — headache, fever, tiredness, gastro-intestinal upset, etc. Stress research pioneer, Dr. Hans Selye, noted that certain *negative emotions* also produced the STH hormone . . . particularly emotions like defeat, futility and discouragement. Here's the point: **Emotional stress can make you "feel" the same way as infectious illness** because the same pituitary hormone is involved. A small increase in STH over a long period of time *may* result in diseases such as asthma, rheumatoid arthritis, high blood pressure, lupus and cancer.

Let's talk about the other pituitary hormone **ACTH**. ACTH acts on the adrenal glands causing them to produce cortisone. Again this happens in response to physical stresses like injuries and infections. But ACTH is also produced by aggressive , unpleasant emotions. This is where the familiar "fight or flight" response comes in. When you've got a bear chasing you out in the woods, your pituitary sends ACTH to the adrenals to get them to pump out the hormones necessary for you to run . . . or, if you decide not to run, to stand and fight. That's the "fight or flight" response.

The trouble is a lot of people constantly experience the "fight or flight" response due to *ongoing* low levels of aggressive, unpleasant emotions. When you're running from that wild animal or stand and fight it, your adrenal hormones do their thing for a few minutes and **then it's over.** The exercise and increased circulation dissipate the hormones so they don't damage you. But when you work in a job or other situation where the stress is ongoing, where you **don't** get to run away or physically fight, the ACTH activity on the adrenals does major damage. Common diseases produced by the ACTH hormone activity include peptic ulcers, some diabetes, and heart disease.

ACTH and STH hormones work in opposition to each other. When ACTH production goes up in response to a "fight or flight" situation, or emotional stress, the effects of the STH hormone are shut down, *including the defense against infection.* Sickness is more likely since the emotional stress is altering your usual immune system response.

"SAD" AND "MAD" DISEASES

We tend to end up with two categories of emotionally induced illness — "sad" diseases and "mad" diseases. The "sad" emotions produce the STH hormone and may result in diseases like arthritis, lupus and cancer. The "mad" diseases produce the ACTH hormone and may result in diseases like ulcers, diabetes, and heart disease. The "sad" diseases eat away on the inside, while the "mad" diseases typically manifest by blowing up on the outside.

Most people can be classified as either predominantly a "sad" personality type or a "mad" personality type. The "sad" type is more introverted, likes solitude, is drained by being around a lot of people, is moody, tends to hold feelings in, can be extremely creative musically or artistically, and *outwardly* doesn't show much difference emotionally from one time to another. The "mad" personality type is generally extroverted, likes being around other people, is a social success, comes across as being positive and energetic, and is very outward in expressing their feelings and opinions. Cancer is perhaps the classic "sad" disease and heart disease is the classic "mad" disease.

STRESS CATEGORIES

I want to look at seven common categories of emotional stress, seven of the most common emotional stresses we all experience . . . which in turn may lead to health problems:

1. Judgment and Guilt —Judgment is basically making negative evaluations of others (or of yourself). It's an "I'm right, you're wrong" type of emotion. Judgment results in, or is often associated with, guilt — an emotion of self-condemnation, what has been called the ***cancer of the conscience***. Judgment and guilt have at their root an offense — with judgment, an offense of someone else, and with guilt, an offense you've committed that's eating away at you.

2. Suppressed Anger — This is where you're mad or embittered against someone, but you don't express it. The anger is buried but eating away at you inside. Christians commonly suppress anger, since we feel it's unspiritual to show anger.

3. Rejection —You don't feel approved of or accepted by others. People communicate to you that you're not OK . . . people like your parents, spouse, children, or so-called "friends."

4. Low Self-Esteem —Perhaps one of the most destructive of all emotional stress categories, this is a feeling of personal unworthiness — a negative, unloving attitude toward yourself.

5. Overwhelmed —Many people are "buried with burden," surrounded by circumstances that are more than they can handle, making them feel unable to perform to expectations.

6. Frustration —This is the stress of contrary experiences — the feeling that things just aren't going according to plan.

7. Deep-Rooted Fear —Finances, marriage, children, or job problems can produce this "what will happen if" emotional stress.

NUTRITIONAL ANSWERS TO STRESS

Nutrition, or any other *physical* treatment is not the answer to the root causes of *emotional* stress. However, it can **help your body cope with emotional stress** while you're working on the root causes. Supplementation that can help on this level includes B-Complex, calcium and magnesium, adrenal glandulars, GABA, and relaxing herbs like Valerian, Scullcap, and Passion Flower.

BIBLICAL ANSWERS TO STRESS

As we approach resolving the above seven areas of emotional stress, note that the first four concern **your view of other people and yourself**, while the last three concern **your view of your circumstances**. May I submit to you the idea that if you adopt the correct view of yourself, others, and your circumstances, you can resolve virtually any kind of emotional stress? I've found two basic principles from the Bible that do just that. The first relates to your view of yourself and others, while the second concerns your view of your circumstances. They are perhaps the two greatest doctrines in all the Bible:

1. Grace —Grace means "unmerited favor," getting something that you don't deserve. The ultimate expression of God's grace is the Cross of Christ, where the price for the sin of his children was paid. All sin for every person must be paid as an expression of God's perfect judgment. Those who trust in Christ are not judged for their sin because Christ was already judged in their place. Those not in Christ will face God's judgment for their sin without Christ as their substitute. Either way, **judgment is out of our hands.** When we judge others or have suppressed anger or feel guilty for already confessed sin, we're failing to accept God's resolution.

The Cross also relates to rejection and approval need. The only person you *have* to have the approval of is God, and you already have that based on His grace. If we're hung up on having to have someone else's approval, we're making that person a god in our life — that's idolatry. The Cross frees us from the need to "perform" for others, since all the ultimately important "performing" was done for us by Christ on the Cross.

What about low self-esteem? The foundation for having a positive self-esteem is **seeing yourself the same way God sees you.** God sees you through his grace, through the complete penalty already paid for you by Christ. If you really embrace what happened at the Cross, there's no legitimate basis for having a low self-esteem.

2. Sovereignty —Understanding the Sovereignty of God releases us from the three remaining stress areas — feeling overwhelmed, frustration and deep-rooted fear. When the Bible says that God is sovereign, it's saying that He's in control, that nothing ultimately goes on without his permission. The way I like to put it is to say that He's behind every circumstance, working as Romans 8:28 says, "All things work together for good, to those who love Him and are called according to His purpose." That means if you love Him and are called according to his purpose, nothing *ultimately* bad can happen to you. God is in control making all circumstances for the believer ultimately good. Trust Him and be stress-free.

Chapter 10

Spiritual Roadblocks to Health

For this reason many among you are weak and sick . . . (I Corinthians 11:30)

Our total health involves physical, mental and spiritual ingredients. Deficiencies in any of those dimensions can rob us of the health God intends. We've already looked at numerous physical and emotional factors of health and now turn to the spiritual. Unfortunately, that's the last place we often look for the roadblock. There is a tendency to either "spiritualize" all ill health or to "naturalize" it. Physical, natural ingredients like nutrition, exercise, sunlight, rest, etc. are mandatory health ingredients. But likewise, emotional and spiritual issues play a major, often deciding role in the health we experience.

BROKEN BY GOD'S LAWS

There's an old saying that, "We don't break God's laws; they break us." That's really just a paraphrase of Galatians 6:7:

> *Do not be deceived, God is not mocked; for whatever a man sows, this he will also reap.*

God has a "way" in all things that is distinct from man's way, a way of life versus the way of death (Proverbs 12:28 and 14:12). Because God is committed to our maturing, ill-health caused by *not* walking in His ways is one *possible* means of correction. Physical sickness may be caused by unresolved spiritual issues both in the Christian and the non-Christian. If you have received Christ and therefore are His child, however, you are *not* being "punished" by sickness, but you may be "chastened" by it:

> *My son, do not regard lightly the discipline of the Lord, nor faint when you are reproved by Him; for those whom the Lord loves, He disciplines, and He scourges every son whom He receives.* (Hebrews 12:5-6)

I find it awesome and exciting that God will use whatever situation necessary to bring me to the lifestyle He has planned—even physical sickness! And He is relentless in His pursuit – you may fight Him, but you will never win. God will never be defeated by our rebellious will.

TEST YOURSELF SPIRITUALLY

Paul wrote to the frequently rebellious Corinthians:

> *Test yourselves to see if you are in the faith; examine yourselves.* (II Corinthians 13:5a)

That counsel is repeated in what is probably the most familiar passage in Scripture of "health chastening" for spiritual causes:

> *Therefore whoever eats the bread or drinks the cup of the Lord in an unworthy manner shall be guilty of the body and blood of the Lord. But let a man examine himself, and so let him eat of the bread and drink of the cup. For he who eats and drinks, eats and drinks judgment to himself, if he does not judge the body rightly. For this reason many among you are weak and sick, and a number sleep. But if we judged ourselves rightly, we should not be judged. But when we are judged, we are disciplined by the Lord in order that we may not be condemned along with the world.* (I Corinthians 11:27-32)

Now you've probably heard that passage read hundreds of times before taking communion at church. It is used as a text to warn non-Christians in church not to take the elements (and that is correct), but is there something more to it? What does it really mean to celebrate the Lord's Supper in an "unworthy manner," to "not judge the body" rightly?

Communion is a remembrance of the Cross and what was accomplished there for us. There are some implications of the Cross that God wants to be a *reality in our lives* before taking the Lord's Supper. Two basic points stand out that might be remembered by the vertical arm and the horizontal arm of the Cross. First, the vertical arm symbolizes the restoration of our relationship with God. This aspect of the Cross tells us that *we are forgiven of sin, but not given license to walk in it.* To profess to be a Christian, celebrate communion, but simultaneously walk in sin is to split in Jesus' face, to re-crucify Him:

> *If we say we have fellowship with Him and yet walk in the darkness, we lie and do not practice the truth; but if we walk in the light as He Himself is in the light, we have fellowship with one another, and the blood of Jesus His Son cleanses us from all sin.* (I John 1:6-7)

> *The one who says, "I have come to know Him," and does not keep His commandments, is a liar, and the truth is not in him; but whoever keeps His word, in him the love of God has truly been perfected. By this we know that we are in Him: the one who says he abides in Him ought himself to walk in the same manner as He walked.* (I John 2:4-6)

If you're a Christian, and there is an area of unconfessed sin in your life, whether in honesty, morality, relationship with others or whatever, taking the Lord's Supper can be as physically dangerous for you as for an unbeliever. It can result in sickness, and in a more extreme case of refusing to repent, premature death may occur.

The second aspect of the Cross, as represented by the horizontal arm, symbolizes the restoration and healing of our relationships with others because of Christ's sacrifice. Just as the horizontal arm of the Cross depends on the vertical arm for its support, so *the restoration of our relationship with God makes possible the restoration of our relationships with other people.* Because we are forgiven by God's grace, we in turn can extend that forgiveness to others. Are you still carrying around a resentment or wounded spirit for someone who wronged you in the past? If so, *don't celebrate the Lord's Supper, lest your health be affected.* Again John writes:

> *The one who says he is in the light and yet hates his brother is in darkness until now.* (I John 2:9)

Or as Jesus put it:

> *If therefore you are presenting your offering at the altar, and there remember that your brother has something against you, leave your offering there before the altar, and go your way; first be reconciled to your brother, and then come and present your offering.* (Matthew 5:23-24)

In the Church age the equivalent to "leaving your offering before the altar" would be *not* taking Communion.

Who has wronged you that you haven't forgiven? Who are you not a peace with? Parents? In-laws? Other relatives? Spouse or former spouse? Children? Employer? Fellow employees? Business associate? Pastor? Friends? Whoever it is, forgive them and/or ask their forgiveness that the Cross may bring healing to your life physically and spiritually. Then you can celebrate the Lord's Supper without it causing health problems.

SEX AND HEALTH

Misuse of sex, I'm convinced, is one of the most frequent spiritual causes of health problems. God's way in sex is simply – *one man with one woman in marriage for life.* Anything outside that invites His chastening, often through physical health problems. Exceptions to this would of course be death of a spouse or biblically valid divorce with subsequent remarriage.

There are several common perversions of God's way in sex that may result in health problems:

1. Fornication – Unmarried people having sex; living together without being married. (See Galatians 5:19-21, I Corinthians 6:18, I Thessalonians 4:3)

2. Adultery – Married person(s) having sex outside of marriage. (See Exodus 20:14, Romans 13:9)

3. Homosexuality – People of the same sex having sexual relations. (See Romans 1:26-27, I Corinthians 6:9-10, I Timothy 1:9-10)

So what are the physical health results of these practices that are so very common in our culture?

Fornication and adultery can lead to various sexually transmitted diseases – syphilis, gonorrhea, herpes, etc. While antibiotics have eliminated much of the threat (and fear) of syphilis and gonorrhea, medical science currently offers no cure for herpes. Then, there's AIDS, likewise without cure, and affecting more and more heterosexual people. Personally, I'm convinced that God can raise up new diseases to discipline mankind into following His ways faster than scientists can develop symptomatic cures.

These more serious sexually transmitted diseases are not the only health problems resulting from violating God's way in sex, however. Vaginal yeast infections are much more common outside of marriage than they are inside of marriage. I have even seen cases where overweight problems correlated with illicit sexual activity – and no amount of diet and nutritional supplementation helped. (Note: I would hasten to add that while fornication and adultery *can* produce weight problems and yeast infections, the reverse is not necessarily true – I'm *not* saying that if you have those health problems, they were produced by sexual sins.)

Then there's homosexuality. The old sexually transmitted diseases are still frequent results, but again God has raised up a new disease to afflict those who violate not only his moral law, but nature itself through homosexuality – AIDS, or Acquired Immune Deficiency Syndrome. AIDS is not just a homosexual disease anymore, but the great majority of cases involve someone who either is homosexual or has had sexual relations with someone who is homosexual. According to some news reports, AIDS has at least resulted in less polygamous homosexuality in favor of more monogamous relationships. Could it be that God is really doing something through this malady, that indeed He is not mocked?

DIVORCE AND HEALTH

Divorce may be a spiritual cause of ill health. Divorce is epidemic among non-Christians, but now the statistics are virtually the same for Christians as well. A close friend shared with me her observation of people switching from the married couples' Sunday School class at her nationally known evangelical church to the singles' class upon dissolution *and even before dissolution* of their marriages! Can there be any wonder at the resulting health problems among Christians who have accepted the world's view of marriage and divorce rather than the Bible's?

Is there such a thing as a "biblically valid divorce?" Bible scholars hold varying views. Jesus' teaching on the subject is pretty blunt:

> . . . *but I say to you that everyone who divorces his wife, except for the cause of unchastity, makes her commit adultery, and whoever marries a divorced woman commits adultery.* (Matthew 5:32)

> *And I say to you, whoever divorces his wife, except for immorality, and marries another woman commits adultery.* (Matthew 19:9)

> *Whoever divorces his wife and marries another woman commits adultery against her, and if she herself divorces her husband and marries another man, she is committing adultery.* (Mark 10:11-12)

> *Everyone who divorces his wife and marries another commits adultery; and he who marries one who is divorced from a husband commits adultery.* (Luke 16:18)

In Paul's writings Christ's teaching is echoed, yet with helpful interpretation:

> *For a married woman is bound by law to her husband while he is living; but if her husband dies, she is released from the law concerning her husband. So then, if while her husband is living, she is joined to another man, she shall be called an adulteress; but if her husband dies, she is free from the law, so that she is not an adulteress, though she is joined to another man.* (Romans 7:2-3)

Paul wrote these words in the context of how Christians have died to the Old covenant law and become "married" to a new "husband," the New Covenant in Jesus Christ. To understand the biblical view of marriage and divorce, we must first understand that marriage is a covenant. A covenant is a "till death do us part" agreement, just as in our traditional marriage ceremonies.

But *physical* death is not necessarily required to terminate a covenant. A covenant in Scripture is also terminated by a *symbolic* or covenantal death. In the Mosaic Law certain crimes were capital offenses such as murder, adultery, homosexuality, bestiality, and others. Many times the actual physical execution was not carried out, yet the person would be considered *covenantally dead* nevertheless. In other words, from God's point-of-view they are dead to His covenant.

For this reason two of the above passages mention *exceptions* of sexual immorality under which divorce is allowable. The covenant was no longer binding because the immoral person was dead *covenantally*. (For further study on this subject I highly recommend Dr. Ray Sutton's book, *Second Chance: Biblical Principles of Divorce and Remarriage*).

While there are thus situations under which divorce appears to be biblically possible (though not required), **most divorces do not take place for these reasons anyway!** The more typical situation is two people who just decide they can't get along with each other anymore. The "I just can't go on any longer" divorce is clearly contrary to God's Word by any honest interpretation. Such an unscriptural divorce is a sin against God's way in marriage and can result in stubborn health problems. If you've gone through an unscriptural divorce, simply confess that to God and receive His forgiveness, just as with any other kind of sin. I believe that any spiritual roadblock to health that was created by your divorce can then be removed.

MARRIAGE AND HEALTH

Just as an unscriptural divorce can produce health problems, so can an unscriptural marriage do similarly. To the husband I would ask:

1. Are you loving your wife as yourself? (Ephesians 5:25-30)

2. Are you living with her in an understanding way? (I Peter 3:7)

3. Are you free from bitterness toward your wife? (Colossians 3:19)

To the wife, I would ask simply:

1. Are you submitting to your husband as to the Lord?

(Colossians 3:18, I Peter 3:1-6, Ephesians 5:22-24)

If these basic instructions from the Lord for our marriages are not being needed, God may use physical health problems to get our attention and force us to straighten out some spiritual issues.

PARENTS AND HEALTH

God's commandment regarding parents in the Scripture also has direct health implications:

> *Children, obey your parents in the Lord, for this is right. Honor your father and mother (which is the first commandment with a promise), that it may be well with you, and that you may live long on the earth.* (Ephesians 6:1-3)

In evaluating someone's health, a negative, resentful attitude toward parents is a major red flag. Sometimes the problem is basic rebellion against their authority, leading to resentment and even outright hatred. Many of my clients have negative feelings toward a parent because of receiving physical, sexual, or emotional abuse as a child that in turn created deep wounds and fear. I've had clients of similar home backgrounds characterized by physical abuse, react in opposite ways with their health problems – one being very thin and wasting away while the other becomes overweight as a defensive barrier against relationships.

God didn't say to honor your parents *if* they were good, righteous and godly. He just said to honor your parents, period. Honoring them doesn't mean they're right in all they do; rather it simply means you respect them as God's chosen parents for you. Even the most wicked parents have been chosen by God for His own purposes in our lives, whether we immediately understand His reasons or not.

THE WORKMAN AND HIS TOOLS

How can you have a positive attitude toward negative things such as an abusive parental situation? Though the remaining chapters cover this question in more detail, let me share one helpful insight. All the circumstances and relationships in your life are but tools God is sovereignly using to mold you into His image. He chooses the tools for His own reasons. He chose my parents, my wife's parents, and a host of other "unchangeables" for His particular design in my life. How can I resent the tools God as the Master Workman chose to construct me with?

Basically, we don't want God to work on us with a crude, rusty, dirty tool. We would prefer a small, shiny, surgical stainless steel, precision-sharpened tool instead – one just to touch up some rough edges. The issue is not what kind of tools are used, but rather who the workman is and how skilled he is. The issue of life is not what kind of parents or any other circumstances you had, but rather God's skill in choosing and using those circumstances as "tools" to bring about His purposes in your life. In skilled hands the crudest tool produces the most beautiful creations. In unskilled hands the finest tool is of little value. You can count on the "skilled hands" of God.

I asked a client if she could see her hostile, abusive father as a tool chosen by God as the Master Workman, for a special purpose in her life. She had never thought of it that way, just as I hadn't previously thought of certain people and situations in my life that way. You see, if you're fighting them, if you're rebelling or resenting, you're really just resisting God and His desired work in your life. And your health, as well as the absence of other forms of prosperity, may be the tools that God uses to drive you to repentance. When I saw my parents and my wife's parents in this way, the resentments, the wounds, the pain, the frustration disappeared. A spiritual issue that had been blocking God's intended blessing on my life had been resolved. This same principle could apply to any relationship or circumstance that God has brought into your life as well.

There are spiritual roadblocks to health, just as there are physical and emotional causes for health problems. Apart from fully submitting to God and the principles of His Word for all of life, total health is impossible. While much of our ill-health admittedly comes from improper physical and nutritional habits, spiritual issues as we discussed can have a direct bearing as well. If you will take the time to meditate on God's Word, allowing Him to bring you into conformity with His way of life in all things, many roadblocks to health and well-being will be removed:

> *My son, give attention to my words, incline your ear to my sayings. Do not let them depart from your sight; keep them in the midst of your heart. For they are life to those who find them, and health to all their whole body.* (Proverbs 4:20-22)

Chapter 11

Defeating Spiritual Strongholds

Neither give place to the devil. (Ephesians 4:27, KJV)

When Christians contemplate their health problems, they tend to gravitate toward one of two extremes: (1) *All my health problems are physical,* **or** (2) *All my health problems are spiritual.* The truth of the matter is that while our health problems are usually physically caused, they can sometimes be spiritually caused.

In the first extreme, someone with obvious emotional and/or spiritual problems, will keep trying vitamin after vitamin hoping the next "wonder product" they try will finally solve their problem. In the second extreme, someone will believe that diet, natural medicines, or even conventional medicines are not the answer, but only faith and prayer. This view is often seen in adherents to the "word-faith" and "deliverance" movements. Let's look at the biblically balanced approach to spiritual issues that most definitely can affect your health — the issue of *spiritual strongholds.*

WHAT IS A "SPIRITUAL STRONGHOLD?"

A spiritual stronghold might be identified as:

> *An area in which we have surrendered "spiritual ground" to Satan, and from which Satan can attack our lives.*

So then, what is "spiritual ground?" "Ground" refers to **jurisdiction**. A little biblical history: When Adam and Eve surrendered to Satan's temptation, jurisdiction over the earth was transferred to Satan. This was obviously still true at the beginning of Jesus' ministry when Satan offered to give Jesus all the kingdoms of the world if He would only fall down and worship him (Matt. 4:8-9).

The Good News is that through Christ's death and resurrection, Satan has been defeated and his kingdom is under judgment (John 16:8-11). Though Satan's *authority* has been removed, his *presence* has not, and will not be removed until the final judgment. Thus, we have a new King—Jesus—in heaven in authority over the earth, and yet there is a lot of previously "surrendered ground" on earth that must *progressively* be taken back by believers in their own lives, as well as in the societies they live in.

But this isn't *just* a matter of ground surrendered by Adam or ground surrendered by ourselves *before* we became Christians. Any Christian can surrender jurisdiction to Satan in any area of his life, thus giving "ground" or a "place" of authority to him. This prompts the scriptural admonition: *". . . and do not give the devil a place (ground)"* (Eph. 4:27).

With each surrender, Satan is given more authority to control your mind, will and emotions. In this situation we become more and more spiritually defeated, *even in seemingly unrelated areas.* We become disillusioned as we sin, confess, repent only to fail again and again. **We fail to understand that the "surrendered ground" provided a place for Satan to build a "stronghold" from which to attack other areas of our lives. Even physical health problems may result.**

SYMPTOMS OF "SPIRITUAL STRONGHOLDS"

So how do you know if you are suffering from "surrendered ground" and "spiritual strongholds?" Here are some common symptoms:

1. Extreme mood changes —Depressive mood swings for no apparent physical reason.

2. Repeated night terrors —More intense and alarming than nightmares.

3. Addiction to rock music —especially heavy metal.

4. Compulsive behavior —usually involving sensual appetites such as food (gluttony, binging, anorexia, bulimia), sex (premarital sex, extra-marital sex, masturbation, homosexuality), drugs, etc.

5. Isolation from family — extended time alone.

6. Involvement in occult games —*Dungeons and Dragons,* addicting and time-consuming computer games.

7. Continual fantasizing —Mentally fulfilling roles of evil.

8. Strange friends —Companionship with those who are in bondage.

9. Extremely negative self-image —Bondage to bizarre fads.

10. Preoccupation with the color black —Black clothing and fingernail polish.

11. Persistent thoughts of suicide —Feeling that there is no hope for the future.

TWO ROOT CAUSES

While there are numerous potential ways someone might develop a spiritual stronghold problem, perhaps the two areas that most often invite Satan to set up shop are **(1) Bitterness** and **(2) Sexual Immorality.**

When you are wronged by someone — a parent, spouse, sibling, co-worker, employee, employer, friend, or whomever — you open the door for Satan to establish a stronghold from which to torment you in other areas, such as depression, uncontrolled anger, lust, eating disorders, or some other physical symptom.

The same is true with sexual immorality. This area especially illustrates how Christians get drawn into the world's way of thinking and living. The world says, "If it feels good, do it" and "Marriage is not required for sex." I understand the unregenerate person believing these lies. But I am saddened, almost to tears, with the Christians that have been drawn into such deception.

Sexual relations outside the bond of marriage, like bitterness, can open the door for all manner of emotional and physical health problems. One that's especially interesting is recurrent vaginal yeast infections, as mentioned in the previous chapter. I've noted over the years that this problem happens a lot more often with women having sex outside of marriage than it does with monogamous married women. I would again repeat: *"We don't break God's laws; God's laws break us."*

TAKING BACK "SURRENDERED GROUND"

Spiritual strongholds, like most problems, are fixable. Here are some steps:

1. Confirm that you are a child of God —The fact that God created you doesn't make you His child. John 1:12 says, *"But as many as received Him* [Christ], *to them He gave the right to become children of God."*

SUGGESTED PRAYER RESPONSE: *"Heavenly Father, I recognize that I am incapable of saving myself and am deserving of eternal separation from You. But I believe on the Lord Jesus Christ for my salvation from sin and from Satan. Amen."*

2. Renounce the Works and Ways of Satan — Christ came not only to save us from the *penalty* of sin in the hereafter, but from the *power* of sin in the here and now. The Bible describes in I John 2:15-17 the "world system" through which Satan operates as consisting of the lust of the flesh, the lust of the eyes, and the boastful pride of life. In *any* area of life we can choose God's way or Satan's way.

SUGGESTED PRAYER RESPONSE: *"Dear Father, I acknowledge that I have been deceived by Satan, who is the father of lies* (John 8:44)*, and that I have also deceived myself by pursuing the lust of the flesh, the lust of the eyes, and the boastful pride of life. I hereby renounce and turn from all of the works and ways of Satan and open my whole life up to the searching eyes of a holy God. Amen."*

3. Commit yourself to the truth at any cost — We defeat Satan's deceptions by agreeing with the truth of God's Word: *"If you abide in My word, then you are truly disciples of Mine; and you shall know the truth, and the truth shall make you free."* (John 8:31-32).

SUGGESTED PRAYER RESPONSE: *"Heavenly Father, I hereby commit myself to learn and obey Your truth, even though it may seem contrary to my natural inclinations. Amen.*

4. Affirm your "position" in Christ — The biblical term "in Christ" refers to the fact that through Christ's death, burial, resurrection, and ascension, Satan has no legal authority over those trusting in Christ's work for their salvation. It is from our "position in Christ" that we hold or surrender "ground" to Satan.

SUGGESTED PRAYER RESPONSE: *"Dear Father, I believe that I am now seated with Christ in the Heavenlies (Eph. 2:8). I am a member of Christ's body and take my position of victory over Satan and all principalities and powers (Col. 2:10) through the death, burial, and resurrection of Christ. Amen."*

5. Recognize and deal with all bitterness —

SUGGESTED PRAYER RESPONSE: *"Heavenly Father, I acknowledge God's mercy that led me to repentance (Rom. 2:4). I ask, Lord, that You would bring to my remembrance those to whom I have not extended your forgiveness. Amen."*

List names as God brings them to mind, including resentment toward yourself or God. Then, one-by-one, state: *"I now forgive (name) for* (state specifically how this person offended you). Then destroy the list.

6. Confess how you have hurt others — Guilt provides ground for Satan to build strongholds. True, appropriate guilt occurs when our conscience convicts our mind and spirit that we have offended God or some other person. Guilt is removed by confessing our offenses to God **and** to the person offended, asking for forgiveness.

SUGGESTED PRAYER RESPONSE: *"Dear Father in Heaven, I purpose to make a list of those whom I have offended as You bring their names to remembrance. I will write down how I offended each person and work out a specific plan to make things right. Amen.*

7. Turn all rebellion into obedience — In I Samuel 15:23 we read the relationship between rebellion and satanic strongholds: *". . . for rebellion is as the sin of witchcraft . . ."* Refusing to recognize God-appointed authorities (parents, husband, pastor, employer, etc.) in our lives causes us to surrender spiritual ground.

SUGGESTED PRAYER RESPONSE: *"Dear Lord, show me where I have not been submissive to your authorities, whom You desire to work through. Amen."*

8. Confess specific sins of the flesh — In I John 1:9 we're instructed to confess specific sins to experience God's cleansing and forgiveness.

SUGGESTED PRAYER RESPONSE: *"Heavenly Father, You have told me to make no provision for the flesh and its lusts* (Rom. 13:14). *I acknowledge that I have given in to fleshly lusts which wage war against my soul* (I Pet. 2:11)."

9. Acknowledge the sins of your ancestors — Even though we are not *responsible* for the sins of our forefathers, or required to confess their sins, their sins *do* affect our lives. Just as Adam passed on a sin nature, so demonic strongholds can be passed from one generation to another, as stated in Exodus 20:5: *". . . for I the Lord thy God am a jealous God, visiting the iniquity of the fathers upon the children unto the third and fourth generation of those that hate Me."*

SUGGESTED PRAYER RESPONSE: *"Father, as your child purchased with Christ's blood, I reject and disown all the sins of my ancestors and cancel out all the demonic working that has been passed from them to me. I now command every familiar spirit and every enemy of the Lord Jesus Christ that is in me or around me to go to the place where Jesus Christ sends them. I do this in the name and authority of the Lord Jesus Christ. Amen.*

10. Rededicate your body to the Lord — Failure to rededicate ourselves to God once the previously surrendered ground has been reclaimed gives Satan continued jurisdiction, as taught in the parable of the unclean spirit leaving and then bringing back seven others more wicked than itself (Matt. 12:43-45). There's no neutral ground here — either we're totally dedicated to Christ, or by default, Satan controls our mind, will and emotions.

SUGGESTED PRAYER RESPONSE: *"Dear Father, I dedicate my body as a living sacrifice to God, and I yield all the members of my body as instruments of righteousness for the Lord and His Kingdom. Amen."*

WELCOME TO TRUE FREEDOM!

Chapter 12

Total Health at the Cross

By His scourging we are healed (Isaiah 53:5c, NASB)

We get sick from the inside out. The progression of sickness, I am convinced, starts with spiritual deficiency, which leads to emotional deficiency, which ultimately leads to physical health problems. Conversely, spiritual wholeness leads to emotional wholeness which leads to physical wholeness.

Now you may think, "Wait a minute; my physical sickness isn't caused by a spiritual deficiency. I'm a believer; I'm saved; I'm Spirit-filled; I've surrendered my life to Christ. What could be wrong with my spiritual perspective?"

If you're sick, I'll tell you what's wrong. Some very important spiritual truths you know in your head have not been applied in your heart as they relate to emotional and physical health. I'm not theorizing here. Client after client coming through our clinics have proved this to me. Though most are Christians and know the Scripture, they had never seen the Cross of Christ applied as I'm about to relate.

WHAT HAPPENED AT THE CROSS?

"Jesus died on the Cross for my sin." That's right, but there's a little more to it than that often incomprehensible statement alone. First of all, He *became* sin before He died for it (II Corinthians 5:21, Romans 8:3, Galatians 3:13). That is, He was totally identified with our sin – past, present and future – on the Cross. All of our human failings, inadequacies, and imperfections were heaped upon Jesus Christ at that one moment in history. So total was His identification with sin that God the Father *had* to turn His back on the Son causing Him to cry out, "My God, My God, why have you forsaken me?" At that one dark moment God judged *all* the sin of those Christ came to save *forever*, poured out His wrath on it, and was satisfied with the shed blood penalty paid by Christ according to His Law (Hebrews 9:22, Leviticus 17:11).

On the Cross Jesus' final words were, "It is finished" (John 19:30). Well, what was finished? It was His mission of paying the penalty for our sin – His work of eliminating the barrier of sin between us and God. Because God is totally just, all sin must be paid for. If you have trusted Christ, your sin is paid for at the Cross – it *is* finished – and you stand forever justified before God. On the other hand, if you have not trusted in Christ, if you are not one of the sheep he came to redeem (John 10:7-16), you will pay for your own sin in eternity – a thought horrible beyond imagination. But either way God's righteous wrath will be satisfied against every sin.

BACK TO YOUR HEALTH

So what in the world does all this theology have to do with health? The truths of the Cross I've just shared, *when applied*, can liberate you from many emotional stresses and resultant health problems. The bottom-line is this: *If you are in Christ, all that is inadequate in you has already been taken care of at the Cross.* All of your sin, all of your imperfection, all of your "missing the mark" is no longer the issue. Consider how these truths of the Cross relate to specific emotional stresses:

1. Judgment – In my clinical experience this is the root of most emotional stress. To judge is to negatively evaluate, to put someone down (others or oneself), to say in effect, "I'm right, therefore you're wrong." Judgment is always based on an offense – someone has blown it, they've "done us dirt," so we judge them. Whether the judgment of believers' sins at the Cross, or the judgment of unbelievers' sins in eternity, one point is clear – God is the Judge of sin, not me. The grace we receive at the Cross allows us to release others from judgment, knowing that is God's job.

2. Guilt – Guilt is the flip side of judgment. It is the emotional stress felt by the one who commits the offense. But if you are in Christ and therefore that offense has been paid for, how can there be legitimate guilt? How can you as a Christian feel legitimately guilty about anything when all those offenses were already paid for at the Cross? I tell my clients: "If you feel guilty about anything, you haven't fully comprehended the Cross." Remember that as Paul points out in Romans 6, grace is not a license to sin. Comprehending the Cross is not an invitation to shun wise health habits, for example. Living under 100% grace motivates us to walk closer to the Lord and His Word, not farther away. Christians do sin and need to confess that sin to God (I John 1:9) and to one another (James 5:16). But we confess our sin *not to be forgiven* but to renew the experiencing of our permanent, total forgiveness that has already been provided at the Cross.

3. Anger – Anger is basically another form of judgment and has similarly been eliminated at the Cross. Anger is motivated again by an offense, whether we're angry at someone else or angry at ourselves. We are released from anger by recognizing that God's anger (wrath) was already poured out at the Cross for believers. Likewise it's God's unique responsibility to express his anger on those whose sin is not paid for by Christ at the Final Judgment. Why insist upon doing something that's God's job?

4. Negative Self-Image – This emotional stress is really nothing but self-judgment – being down on yourself. If all the inadequacy in you was dealt with at the Cross, what's left to be down on yourself about? When Christ took on all your sin at the Cross, He gave you all His righteousness and perfection in exchange:

He made Him who knew no sin to be sin on our behalf, that we might become the righteousness of God in Him. (II Corinthians 5:21)

What a trade! Now that's how God looks at you – just as He looks at His Son. How about you looking at you that way?

5. Approval Need – Do you feel your emotional stress in others' approval or disapproval? This might be called "reverse judgment." Others find things wrong with you and disapprove. So what? God approves of you because He's already atoned at the Cross for what's lacking in you. Those who disapprove of you are misinformed! Approval from people comes and goes – you can never be sure of having the approval of others. As a matter of fact, the more closely you follow the Lord, the more disapproval you are likely to get. If you depend on others' approval, you're going to live on an emotional roller coaster. However, God's approval of you is unwavering because He's already paid for what is lacking in you at the Cross.

Approval from other people will always be undependable, so why not make a decision to look only to God for approval? That secure foundation will free you from the moment to moment, day to day approval of people. Then when you do receive human approval, it can just be the icing on the cake. Decide that the only approval you really *have* to have is God's, and recognize that, as a redeemed believer, you have that already because of the Cross.

6. Performance Orientation – Being performance oriented refers to basing your self-worth on **what you do** rather than **who you are**. If you feel like you're "measuring up" to whatever standards you've established, you feel pretty good about yourself. But if you're not measuring up, you get really down on yourself. Is there a self-condemning standard constantly whipping you internally to do better and putting you down for poor performance? If so, you know the "performance treadmill" I speak of. 'Tis a cruel master indeed.

Again the Cross frees us from performance and its self-condemnation. Paul wrote:

There is therefore now no condemnation for those who are in Christ Jesus . . . For what the Law could not do, weak as it was through the flesh, God did: sending His own Son in the likeness of sinful flesh and as an offering for sin, He condemned sin in the flesh, **in order that the requirement of the Law might be fulfilled in us**, *who do not walk according to the flesh, but according to the Spirit.* (Romans 8:1, 3-4)

When we look at ourselves *not* based on our performance, our self-image can soar right through the roof? How can I be down on myself when my performance is no longer at issue? God's performance makes us perfect – the absolute perfect standard of the Law *has been fulfilled* in us (Romans 8:4). Do you see yourself as perfect? God does, because of the Cross. This is a good test: If you *don't* see yourself as perfect through the Cross of Christ, that probably indicates you're still living under a performance orientation.

If you're thinking, "Wait a minute! I'm not perfect; I blow it all the time," let me explain further. Yes, we still stumble in our actions – the "what we do" part of our lives. But our actions are no longer the issue. Our actions have been covered, paid for by Christ. Instead of our "who we are" being determined by our actions, it is now determined by Christ's actions as our Substitute. As we focus on this perspective, we allow God's "performance" to flow through us by the power of the Holy Spirit – His strength and power are thus perfected in our weakness.

Several conclusions can be drawn from the Cross that relate directly to emotional and correspondingly physical health:

1. You're OK – As one trusting in Christ, God accepts you just the way you are. None of your trying, doing, or striving can make you more acceptable to Him. All that is imperfect, missing the mark, or in any way inadequate in you has been paid for. You are free. Now I know He isn't finished with maturing you yet, but in His sovereignty you're right on schedule with that growth process. He totally accepts you for who and what and where you are today. How about agreeing with Him? It's guaranteed to change your life!

2. You can escape the performance treadmill – Jesus has done all the performing for you. Base your self-image on who you are, not what you do. Jesus took care of the latter. God isn't at all impressed with your trying. But when you "cease striving and know that He is God" (Psalm 46:10), when you see that your only source of adequacy is the Cross, *then and only then* can He work *His* performance through you by the Holy Spirit. And His performance (unlike your performance) won't destroy your health in the process.

3. The end result is wholeness – spiritually, emotionally, and physically. As I look at Jesus' ministry I see Him only in one business – making people whole. His finished work on the Cross is the foundation for that wholeness in body, mind, and spirit.

Chapter 13

Living in God's Sovereignty

His sovereignty rules over all (Psalm 103:19)

The capstone of experiencing total health is to truly discover God's sovereignty over everything in your life. Nothing excites me more than introducing someone to the concept of the sovereignty of God. It is such a dynamic and life-transforming truth. Like many of the other areas shared in this book, most Christians have not practically applied this truth. To understand the sovereignty of God is to be released from the spiritual and emotional bondage that so often destroys our physical health.

All too often candy-coated Christians and churches (both figuratively and literally) have portrayed a false view of the Christian life, sort of like the Army recruit's version of the Army – why, it's a "bed of roses." It's basically, "Accept Jesus and all your problems will be solved" – blue sky till the sweet by and by. All I can say is if you're honest and if you've been a Christian for very long, you know that's a bunch of baloney! The Christian life often seems (at least from our perspective) more like hell on earth than heaven on earth. Usually, becoming a Christian is the *beginning* of your problems rather than the end of them . . . *and this is by God's design!* Over 45 years of getting knocked around in the Christian life have made me a cold-blooded realist. In the process of being spiritually, emotionally and financially beaten and bloodied repeatedly, however, a funny thing has happened – I've begun to discover the sovereignty of God.

WHAT IS SOVEREIGNTY?

A. W. Tozer in his classic study of the attributes of God, *The Knowledge of the Holy*, says:

God's sovereignty is the attribute by which He rules His entire creation, and to be sovereign God must be all-knowing, all-powerful, and absolutely free.[1]

God's sovereignty refers to His Kingship over His creation. He is in charge. Nothing happens apart from His rule. The Lord is on the throne and He is in control. This is the key: ***He is in ultimate control of every circumstance in your life. When you see God behind everything that happens to you, burdens, frustrations, failures and fears are all dissolved.*** Truly comprehending God's sovereignty eliminates emotional stress!

However, the fact of the matter is that most Christians *don't* see God behind all their circumstances. They may blame their parents, their spouse, their boss, their children, those that have defrauded them, and most of all they blames themselves. They credit everybody and everything with the problems of their lives but God – the One who initiated their problems in the first place.

> *We turn to God for help when our foundations are shaking, only to learn that it is God who is shaking them.* – Charles C. West

> *When suffering comes, we yearn for some sign from God, forgetting we have just had one.* – Mignon McLaughlin, *The Neurotics Notebook*

IS GOD BEHIND *EVERY* CIRCUMSTANCE?

Is your god (small "g" intended) in control of everything that's going on? The God of the Bible is. Does your "god" at times bring death, destruction, poverty and calamity? The God of the Bible does. Did your "god" create wicked people to carry out His purposes? The God of the Bible did. Or is your "god" just doing the "good" things and in effect *sharing* his sovereignty with Satan who is doing the "bad" things?

Unlike the view of most Christians, the Scripture does not portray a "good" God duking it out with an evil god, Satan. That's the dualistic view of Zoroastrianism, not Christianity. Don't misunderstand me. God *is* good (though by *His* definition of goodness not ours) and Satan *is* evil. *But* Satan does no evil toward you apart from God's permission. Psalm 103:19 declares:

> *The Lord has established His throne in the heavens; and His sovereignty rules over all.*

And that "all" includes all of Satan's activity. I loved the way one of my Bible teachers put it years ago, "Satan is just God's messenger boy." Deuteronomy 4:39 reiterates:

> *Know therefore today, and take it to heart, that the Lord, he is God in heaven above and on earth below; there is no other.*

How about Isaiah 45:5-7:

> *I am the Lord and there is no other; besides Me there is no other God . . . The One forming light and creating darkness, causing well-being and creating calamity; I am the Lord who does all these.*

Then there's Proverbs 16:4:

> *The Lord has made everything for His own purpose, even the wicked for the day of evil.*

But does God actually bring death, destruction and poverty? Part of godly Hannah's prayer in I Samuel 2:6-8 reads:

> *The Lord kills and makes alive; He brings down to Sheol and raises up. The Lord makes poor and rich; he brings low, he also exalts. He raises the poor from the dust, He lifts the needy from the ash heap to make them sit with nobles, and inherits a seat of honor; for the pillars of the earth are the Lord's and He set the world on them.*

So often as Christians we are practical deists, as it were, believing God has turned His back on His creation and is really not involved in its moment by moment details. Isaiah tells us he is very much in charge:

> The Lord of hosts has sworn saying, "Surely, just as I have intended so it has happened, and just as I have planned so it will stand . . . This is the plan devised against the whole earth; and this is the hand that is stretched out against all the nations. For the Lord of hosts has planned, and who can frustrate it? And as for his stretched-out hand, who can turn it back?" (Isaiah 14:24, 26-27)

As the prophet Jeremiah pondered the ruins of destroyed Jerusalem at the beginning of the Babylonian Captivity, he acknowledged God's complete sovereignty over the destruction:

> Who is there who speaks and it comes to pass, unless the Lord has commanded it? Is it not from the mouth of the Most High that both good and ill go forth? Why should any living mortal, or any man, offer complaint in view of his sins? (Lamentations 3:37-39)

THE RIGHT TO AFFLICT

What it really gets down to on the very practical level is the question, "Does God really have the right to afflict us with suffering?" Few writers in the Scripture acknowledged this "right" of God more than the writers of the Psalms. The Psalmist confessed in Psalm 119:75:

> I know, O Lord, that Thy judgments are righteous, and that in faithfulness Thou has afflicted me.

In Psalm 71:20 the Psalmist likewise acknowledges God behind his suffering:

> Thou, who has shown me many troubles and distresses, wilt revive me again, and wilt bring me up again from the depths of the earth.

These men of God loved God deeply, yet also knew He was behind their suffering – suffering that had divine purpose. A. W. Tozer beautifully summarizes:

> *God cannot use a man greatly until He first wounds Him deeply.*

Outside of Scripture itself, the deepest statements expounding the sovereignty of God I have ever read come from a Puritan pastor in England named Stephen Charnock, who lived from 1628 – 1680. His book, *The Existence and Attributes of God*, is still considered the greatest classic ever written on God's attributes. Charnock reasons:

> *Affliction is an act of His sovereignty. By this right of sovereignty may not God take way any man's goods since they were His doles? As He was not indebted to us when He bestowed them, so He cannot wrong us when He removes them. He takes from us what is more His own than it is ours, and was never ours but by His gift, and that for a time only, not forever. By this right He may determine our times, put a period to our days when He pleases, strip us of one member, and lop off another. Man's being was from Him, and why should He not have a sovereignty to take what He had a sovereignty to give?*

> *Why should this seem strange to any of us, since we ourselves exercise an absolute dominion over those things in our possession which have sense and feeling, as well as over those that want it? Doth not every man think he hath an absolute authority over the utensils of his house, over his horse, his dog, to preserve, or to kill him, to do what he pleases with him, without rendering any other reason than, "It is my own?" May not God do much more? Doth not His dominion over the works of His hands transcend that which a man can claim over his beast that he never gave life to?*

> *He that dares dispute against God's absolute right, fancies himself as much a god as his creator; understands not the vast difference between the divine nature and his own, between the sovereignty of God and his own.*[2]

Think for a moment about your own emotional stress problems that are causing you burden, frustration, failures or fears. Is it a problem with your spouse, your job, your children, your finances, or your health? Do you see those problems as coming from God or from somewhere else, as part of God's special, wonderful design for your life, or as just "bad breaks?"

THE EXAMPLE OF JOB

Nowhere can we put our trials into perspective with God's sovereignty as in the Book of Job. I remember once a Christian friend, overwhelmed with suffering in his life, angrily sneering at me, "Don't talk to me about Job – as far as I'm concerned he got a raw deal." Is that what you think?

The Book of Job is outstanding in all of Scripture, for in it we see the very curtain of heaven drawn back, allowing us to view the activity of Satan in relationship to God. I often ask my clients, "Who initiated Job's suffering – Satan or God?" Due to the fascination most have with a "devil made me do it" theology, most credit Satan for Job's suffering, though even a quick look at the texts clearly shows God to be the initiator. God "baited" Satan to afflict Job by bragging about Job's blameless character:

> *And the Lord said to Satan, "Have you considered My servant Job? For there is no one like him on earth, a blameless and upright man, fearing God and turning away from evil"* (Job 1:8)

Satan didn't ask permission from God to afflict Job – God suggested it to Satan! In one breath God declared Job to be the most righteous man on earth and encouraged Satan to bring incredible suffering into his life. Do you understand a God like that? Job did, as he confessed, after losing wealth and children:

> *Naked I came from my mother's womb, and naked I shall return there. The Lord gave and the Lord has taken away. Blessed be the name of the Lord.* (Job 1:21)

It says he fell to the ground and *worshipped* when told of his great losses. Is that what you would do? Is that what I would do?

After he was personally afflicted in the next round of trials with boils from head to foot, Job rebuked his unbelieving wife's "curse God and die" suggestion with this:

> *Shall we indeed accept good from God and not accept adversity?* (Job 2:10b)

Not even once in the entire book does Job ever credit Satan with his suffering. He only recognizes God behind it all. That's the first step you need to accomplish – recognize that adversity in your life comes *from God's hand*. The second step though is to see what God is doing in that adversity, to get a perspective on just what His design is.

GOD'S ULTIMATE OBJECTIVE

To understand Job's trials (and our own) we must first understand God's purpose in history. His objective is *not* to give you a nice, fun time. God has only one ultimate objective – to glorify Himself. That's what He was doing in Job's trials and that's what He's doing in yours and mine – and that's all that really matters. When *His* glorification outranks your comfort, not only will you experience relief from emotional stress, but you will enter a new dimension in your Christian maturity.

I appreciate honesty, and I've had some clients get really honest with me at this point and ask, "How can God be so egotistical?" That's really what our attitude tends to be, isn't it? We, in effect, think that He is *our* servant instead of the other way around. What do you have that God hasn't given to you? Therefore, doesn't He have the right to take away what He had a right to give? Is God my debtor? Apart from His grace, His gift of salvation, He owes us only judgment and damnation, and let's not forget it. Romans 9:20-21 makes this clear:

> *On the contrary, who are you, O man, who answers back to God? The thing molded will not say to the molder, "Why did you make me like this," will it? Or does not the potter have a right over the clay, to make from the same lump one vessel for honorable use, and another for common use?*

Stephen Charnock commented on this passage this way:

May not the potter after his labor, either set his vessel up to adorn his house, or knock it in pieces, and fling it upon the dunghill, separate it to some noble use, or condemn it to some sordid service? Is the right of God over His creatures less than that of the potter over his vessel, since God contributed all to His creature, but the potter never made the clay, which is the substance of the vessel, nor the water, which was necessary to make it tractable, but only molded the substance of it into such a shape?

The vessel that is framed, and the potter that frames it, differ only in life; the body of the potter, whereby he executes his authority, is of no better a mold than the clay, the matter of his vessel; shall he have no absolute power over that which is so near him, and shall not God over that which is so infinitely distant from Him?

The vessel perhaps might plead for itself that it was once part of the body of a man, and as good as the potter himself, whereas no creature can plead it was part of God, and as good as God Himself.[3]

GOD'S PURPOSE IN EVIL

It's admittedly hard to see God working in evil. What is His design, His purpose in, as Proverbs 16:4 puts it, "making the wicked for the day of evil?" For God to be sovereign *He must use evil* for His design, in order that it ultimately brings glory to Him. Joseph is a classic example from the Old Testament. Imagine being sold into slavery by your own brothers. Pretty evil, I would say. But who was behind that hideous crime? Years later *Joseph himself stated that God had done it*, that He had superintended Joseph's enslavement and imprisonment using the evil in his brother's hearts to fulfill His divine purpose:

> *And as for you, you meant evil against me, but God meant it for good in order to bring about this present result, to preserve many people alive.* (Genesis 50:20)

All a matter of perspective, isn't it? How do you know that the suffering you're going through is really evil? We got into this whole rhubarb in the first place when Adam and Eve decided to judge good and evil instead of just following the Lord. I'm sure Joseph initially was convinced that his enslavement was the height of evil and that God had surely abandoned him. But somewhere along the line he came to see that *with a sovereign God evil is displaced by divine destiny*. His suffering was but a tool in God's hand to save the nation of Israel and preserve the seed of the coming Messiah. Joseph came to a point of thankfulness for the evil God had taken him through at the hands of his brothers. When he saw the big picture he was emotionally released from anger, judgment, bitterness and frustration. But how about you? Have you learned that same lesson? Have you put your own suffering into the perspective of God's sovereignty?

I hear some pretty gross things from my clients. I hear the stories of childhood beatings and sexual molestation, of infidelity, of drunken rampages, of financial fraud and you name it. No matter what your scar, your emotional healing begins when you come to Joseph's perspective – when you see God in that circumstance, no matter how awful it was. He was and is sovereign and has design in all that happens to you. He is omnipotent and *could have* prevented or delivered you from that trial. But He chose not to. Why? Is He unwilling or disinterested? No, He's just fulfilling His plan instead of yours. And friend, what a privilege it is to participate, to act out our part in His script whether it means comfort or abuse, sickness or health, injury or safety, freedom or prison, poverty or riches, life or death.

MORE THAN SOVEREIGN

There are two basic reactions to discovering God's sovereignty – running to Him in worship or running from Him in rebellion. That's why it's so important to balance God's sovereignty with an understanding of His goodness, grace, love and mercy. Without the Cross God's sovereignty would be terrifying. But the Cross proclaims an almost incomprehensible message – God is so committed to me that in spite of my unworthiness, He died for me. He paid the ultimate price to have a relationship *with me* for eternity! He has proven His love. But have we proven our faith in His love? I can rest in His inescapable sovereign hand leading in my life whether He brings joy or suffering, sickness or health, comfort or pain, blessing or hardship, life or death. That's the perspective Job had when in the midst of losing everything at the hand of the sovereign God he confessed:

> *Though He slay me, yet will I trust Him.* (Job 13:15)

Let me close with a favorite quote from Alan Redpath in his book, *Victorious Christian Living*:

> *There is nothing – no circumstance, no trouble, no testing – that can ever touch me until, first of all it has gone past God and past Christ, right through to me. If it has come that far, it has come with a **great purpose**, which I may not understand at the moment. But as I **refuse** to become panicky, as I lift up my eyes to Him and accept it as coming from the throne of God for some great purpose of **blessing** to my own heart, no sorrow will ever disturb me, no trial will **ever** disarm me, no circumstance will cause me to fret – for I shall **rest in the joy of what my Lord is!** That is the rest of victory.*[4]

I guarantee that perspective will transform your health in body, mind and spirit.

Closing Thoughts

God created you to experience true wholeness of life – in body, mind, and spirit. His mission is to make you whole as He conforms you to the image of His Son, Jesus Christ.

Within our body, mind, and spirit totality, needs vary according to the person. Some have lined up well with the Creator's way in their spiritual redemption, but may be emotional and physical wrecks. Others are mature emotionally but perhaps out of touch physically or spiritually. Many in today's health-conscious society have discovered God's health principles but haven't yet discovered the complete relationship with the One who made those principles.

Whatever state you're in as you finish this book, God wants to meet you and touch you and change you. He wants to fill the "holes in your wholeness." The only question is, "Will you let Him?" Will you dare to let Him invade your life with His transforming truth? Will you receive His truths of total health as just "good views" to never penetrate beyond your intellectual curiosity, or will you let it be "good news" that reaches and touches the heart and will?

The choice is yours.

(If you found this book helpful, will you consider leaving a review? I would very much appreciate it. The review page of this book may be accessed at: **http://www.amazon.com/dp/B00M9TFQKE** and then clicking on "Customer Reviews." Thanks so much! -- *Monte Kline*)

Footnotes

Chapter 1

1. Bodog F. Beck, M.D., *Honey and Health*, Robert M. McBride, New York, 1938, p. 66.

2. Bodog F. Beck, M.D., and Doree Smedley, *Honey and Your Health*, Robert M. McBride, New York, 1944, p. 40.

3. Ibid., p. 35.

4. Ibid., p. 35-36.

Chapter 2

1. OregonLive.com, 11/23/09.

2. Environmental Working Group study at **http://www.ewg.org/tap-water/home**.

3. *International Journal of Cancer* April 15, 2006; 118(8):2040-2047 and Yahoo News May 5, 2006.

4. Richard Mesquita, AquaMD, "The Dirty Little Secret Behind the Chlorine in Your Water," **www.mercola.com**, 3/19/05.

5. National Sanitation Foundation International (NSF). Toxicology and Carcinogenesis Studies of Sodium Fluoride in F344/N Rats and B6C3f1 Mice. Technical report Series No. 383. NIH Publ. No 91-2848. National Institute of Envornomental Health Sciences, Research Triangle Park, NC.

6. Wang C, et. al. (1997). [Changes of coenzyme Q content in brain tissues of rats with fluorosis]. *Zhonghua Yu Fang Yi Xue Za Zhi* 31:330-3.

7. Mahaffey KR, Stone CL. (1976). Effect of High Fluorine (F) intake on Tissue Lead (Pb) Concentrations. *Federation Proceedings* 35:256.

8. Lin FF, et. al. (1991). The relationship of a low-iodine and high-fluorine environmental to subclinical cretinism in Xinjiang. *Iodine Deficiency Disorder Newsletter* Vol. 7. No. 3. **http://www.fluoridealert.org/IDD.htm**.

9. Stecher P, et. al. (1960). The Merck Index of Chemicals and Drugs. Merck & Co., Inc., Rathway NJ. P. 952.

10. Waldbott GL, et. al. (1978). Fluoridation: The Great Dilemma. Coronado Press, Inc. Lawrence, Kansas.

11. Hileman B. (1989). New studies cast doubt on fluoridation benefits. *Chemical and Engineering News* May 8. **http://www.fluoridealert.org/NIDR.htm**.

12. Maupome G, et. al. (2001). Patterns of dental caries following the cessation of water fluoridation. *Community Dentistry and Oral Epidemiology* 29:37-47.

Chapter 3

1. Order *The Sick & Tired Manual* at the following link:

http://www.pacifichealthcenter.com/shop/product-list.php?pg1-cid92.html

2. Julian N. Kenyon, M.D., *21st Century Medicine*, (Wellingsborough, Northamptonshire: Thorsons Publishers Limited, 1986).

3. Hal A. Huggins, D.D.S., *It's All in Your Head*, (Avery, 1993), p. 29, 59.

4. J. H. Tilden, M.D., *Food: Its Influence as a Factor in Disease and Health*, (New Haven: Keats, 1976), p. 1.

5. John A. Schindler, M.D., *How to Live 365 Days a Year*, (New York: Fawcett Crest, 1954), p. 34.

6. Hans Heinrich Reckeweg, M.D., *Homotoxicology*, (Albuquerque: Menaco Publishing, 1980), p. 18-19.

7. Order *The Junk Food Withdrawal Manual* at the following link:

http://www.pacifichealthcenter.com/shop/product-list.php?pg1-cid92.html

Chapter 5

1. "Metop-A Satellite Measures Ozone Hole," **www.theozonehole.com/metop.htm**, October 5, 2007.

2. *American Journal of Public Health*, April 1995; 85; 4:546-550.

3. Holman, Ralph T., et. al., "Omega 3 But Not Omega 6 Fatty Acids Inhibit Ap-1 Activity and Cell Transformation in JB6 Cells," *Proceedings of the National Academy of Sciences*, June 19, 2001, 98:13, 7510-7515.

4. *Cancer Research*, 60(15):4139-45, August 1, 2000.

5. *Archives of Environmental Health*, 1990; 45:261-267.

6. Mercola, Joseph, D.O., "The Sunscreen Myth: How Sunscreen Products Actually Promote Cancer," **www.mercola.com**.

7. *Journal of Investigative Dermatology*, 1980; 75:122-127.

8. *Epidemiology*, 1992; 3)3):263-265.

9. Prota, G., "Recent Advances in the Chemistry of Melanogenesis in Mammals," *Journal of Investigative Dermatology*, 1980; 75:122-127.

10. Rampen, F.H. "Nelewans, R.t., Kerbeek, A. L. M., "Is Water Pollution a Cause of Cutaneous Melanoma?," *Epidemiology*, 1992; 3(3): 263-265.

11. The Walnut Creek Contraceptive Drug Study, US National Institutes of Health, Vol. III, 1986:247-252.

12. Veith, R., "Vitamin D Supplementation, 25-Hydroxyvitamin D Concentrations and Safety," *American Journal of Clinical Nutrition*, 1999; 69:842-856.

13. Veith, R., Chan, P-C R, MacFarlane, G. D., "Efficacy and Safety of vitamin D3 Intake Exceeding the Lowest Adverse Effect Level," *American Journal of Clinical Nutrition*, 2001; 71:288-294.

14. Rostand, S. G., "Ultraviolet Light May Contribute to Geographic and Racial Blood Pressure Differences," *Hypertension*, 1997; 30:150-156.

15. Krause, R., et. al., "Ultraviolet B and Blood Pressure," *Lancet*, 1998; 352:709-710.

16 . Pfeifer, M., et. al., "Effects of a Short-Term Vitamin D3 and Calcium Supplementation on Blood Pressure and Parathyroid Hormone Levels in Elderly Women," *Journal of Clinical Endocrinology*, Metab 2001; 86:1,633-1637.

17. Lind, L., et. al., "Reduction of Blood Pressure During Long-Term Treatment with Active Vitamin D (alphacalcidol) is Dependent on Plasma Renin Activity and Calcium Status. A Double-Blind, Placebo-Controlled Study," *American Journal of Hypertension*, 1989; 2:20-25.

18. Kristal-Boneh, E., et. al., "Association of Calcitriol and Blood Pressure in Normotensive Men," *Hypertension*, 1997; 30:1,289-1,294.

19. Lind, L., et. al., "Vitamin D is Related to Blood pressure and Other Cardiovascular Risk Factors in Middle-Aged Men," *American Journal of Hypertension*, 1995; 2:20-25.

20. Hypponen, E., Laara, E., Reunanen, A., Jarvelin, M.R., Virtanen, S. M., "Intake of Vitamin D and Risk of Type I Diabetes: A Birth-Cohort Study," *Lancet*, 2001; 358(9,292): 1,500 – 1503.

21. Ibid.

22. Adams, Mike, "New Research Shows Vitamin D Slashes Risk of Cancers by 77 Percent; Cancer Industry Refuses to support Cancer Prevention," **http://www.newstarget.com/z021892.html**, June 8, 2007.

23. *American Journal of Epidemiology*, October 12, 2007, as quoted in "Sunbathing Cuts Breast Cancer Risk in Half," **www.mercola.com**.

24. Nutrition & Healing E-Newsletter 7/13/2004.

25. *Proceedings of the National Academy of Sciences*, October 30, 2007; 104; 44:17500-17505.

Chapter 8

1. Spurgeon, Charles, *Morning and Evening*, Nashville: Thomas Nelson, 1994, November 26th morning reading.

About the Author

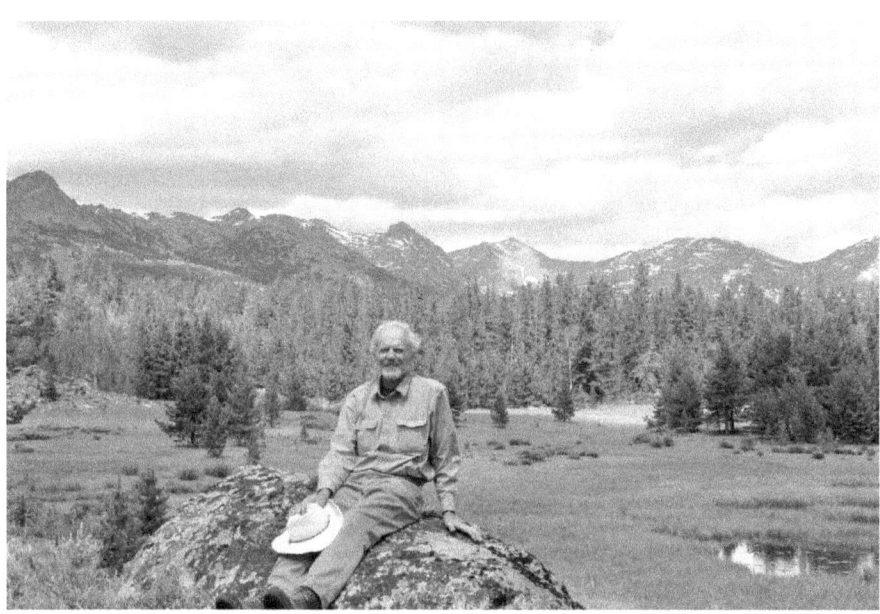

After growing up in the Midwest, Monte Kline came to the Pacific Northwest in pursuit of a college education in geology and to enjoy the region's scenic beauty. However, coming to know Christ his sophomore year changed his plans, redirecting him after graduation into several years of college campus Christian ministry. During that time he developed a serious cancer condition that was ultimately resolved with a natural medicine approach. This experience launched him into a career of speaking, writing books and presenting health and nutrition from a biblical perspective, including *Eat, Drink & Be Ready, The Junk Food Withdrawal Manual, Vitamin Manual for the Confused, The Sick & Tired Manual, Body, Mind & Health* and *Face to Face*. After completing a graduate degree in Nutrition & Wholistic Health Sciences, Monte went into practice as a Clinical Nutritionist in 1984. He currently directs two Pacific Health Center practices in the Northwest.

Monte, along with his wife Nancy live near Sisters, Oregon.

Monte may be contacted regarding speaking engagements or his clinical practice at **drkline@pacifichealthcenter.com** or Pacific Health Center, PO Box 1066, Sisters, OR 97759.

Appendix A – Physical Health

A Health Strategy for Anyone . . . Anywhere

The physical health checklist in *Body, Mind & Health* requires individual screening to assess for "common denominator" factors including:

Food & environmental sensitivities

Nutrient deficiencies

Toxins

Organ stress

Compatible natural remedies

Ultimately, we must have answers to two fundamental questions:

1. What's *missing* in my body (that should be there)?

2. What's *present* in my body (that should not be there)?

Thus, our health approach is then to put the good into the body and remove the bad. But how does one answer those questions? How do you find out "what's missing" and "what's present," so as to free up your body's natural healing processes?

Enter **Remote Health Screening** or what we like to call **E-Health.** Pacific Health Center tests clients, not only at our local Oregon offices, but literally all over the world with our custom designed Zyto technology program featuring:

1. Remote testing through a "Hand Cradle" plugged into your PC computer:

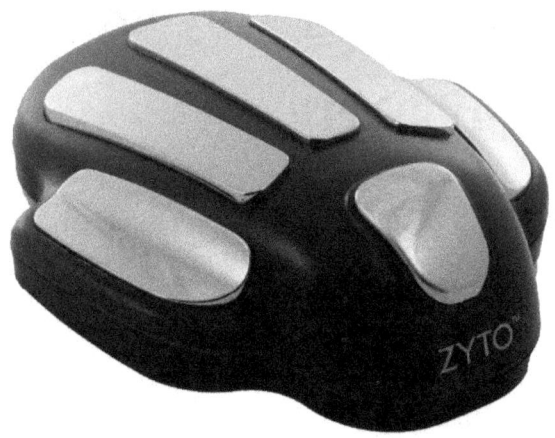

2. Non-invasively measures changes in galvanic skin resistance in response to thousands of "virtual stressors and balancers" – essentially computer signatures that simulate exposure to an item.

3. Assessing "common denominators" of all health problems – food & environmental sensitivities, nutrient deficiencies, toxins, stressed organs, and compatible natural remedies.

4. Remote connection to Pacific Health Center through the internet, while talking by phone or Skype and observing testing computer screen through screen sharing – just as in in the office as shown below:

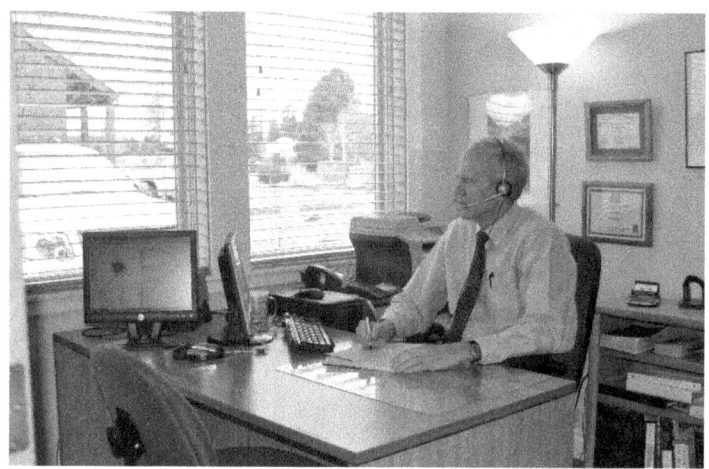

Pacific Health Center's approach, along with a demonstration of the remote, "E-Health" screening, may be viewed in the Free **SICK & TIRED WEBINAR** at the following link:

http://www.pacifichealthcenter.com/client-webinar-signup-recorded.html

You may also schedule a Free Health Screening Telephone Consultation with Monte Kline to discuss your health issues at the following link:

http://www.pacifichealthcenter.com/health-screening.html

We look forward to helping you to better health . . . naturally.

-- Monte Kline, Clinical Nutritionist

Appendix B – Emotional & Spiritual Health

Encounter God through Personal Retreats

Dealing with the "missing ingredients" of *physical health* is one thing, but what about your emotional and spiritual health? How do you bring healing to those areas? My suggestion: Have an **encounter with God** – what I call a **Personal Retreat**.

Has God spoken to you lately? Imagine a whole new way of meeting with God that would transform your Christian life. What if you could create special times alone with God for illumination, direction on decisions, and just the sheer enjoyment of being in His presence . . . like nothing you ever experienced before? What if you could come "face to face" with God? My book, *Face to Face: Meeting God in the Quiet Places* provides the blueprint. Following the pattern of Abraham, Elijah, Paul, and Jesus, *Face to Face* shows the way to create those life-changing encounters. You will discover:

A way to meet with God and hear his voice

Keys to escaping the "noise" and busyness of life

An alternative to "Christmas list" praying

How to "capture" your spiritual transformation

How to encounter God through Personal Retreats

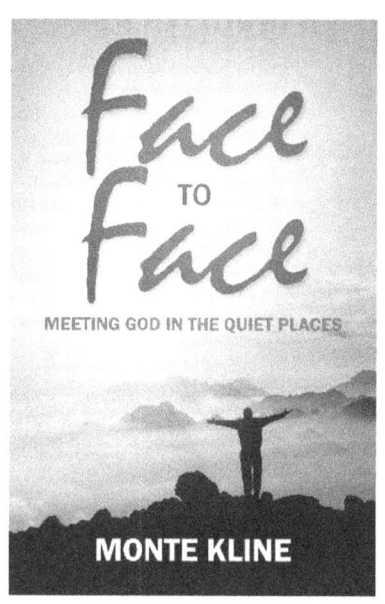

What others say . . .

> ***Face to Face*** *lays out a game plan for a deeper and more meaningful relationship with Christ.* – Tom Flick, Motivational Speaker and former NFL quarterback

> *Only you and Him. It stands to reason you need some quality time **Face to Face.*** – Stu Weber, Author of Tender Warrior

Order at this link: **http://www.amazon.com/dp/B00M1ZBIU8**

www.ingramcontent.com/pod-product-compliance
Lightning Source LLC
Chambersburg PA
CBHW070652290526
45790CB00001B/282